Health Matters

Health Matters

8 Steps That Can Save Your Life—and Your Family's Health

TAYLOR GRANT

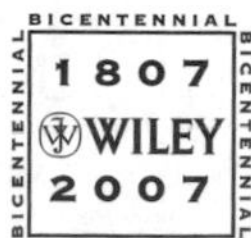

John Wiley & Sons, Inc.

Published by John Wiley & Sons, Inc., Hoboken, New Jersey
Published simultaneously in Canada

Drawings by Ann E. Sabo; copyright © Taylor Grant Enterprises, LLC.

Wiley Bicentennial Logo: Richard J. Pacifico

The information contained in this book is not intended to serve as a replacement for professional medical advice. Any use of the information in this book is at the reader's discretion. The author and the publisher specifically disclaim any and all liability arising directly or indirectly from the use or application of any information contained in this book. A health care professional should be consulted regarding your specific situation.

For general information about our other products and services, please contact our Customer Care Department within the United States at (800) 762-2974, outside the United States at (317) 572-3993 or fax (317) 572-4002.

Wiley also publishes its books in a variety of electronic formats. Some content that appears in print may not be available in electronic books. For more information about Wiley products, visit our web site at www.wiley.com.

Library of Congress Cataloging-in-Publication Data:

Grant, Taylor, date.
Health matters : 8 steps that can save your life—and your family's health / Taylor Grant.
p. cm.
Includes bibliographical references and index.
ISBN: 978-0-470-04572-5 (pbk.)
1. Health. I. Title.
RA776.G775 2007
613—dc22

2007001704

Printed in the United States of America

10 9 8 7 6 5 4 3 2 1

For John, Sam, and Jack:
Thanks for the roller coaster ride, guys.
But then, the carousel's just not our style.

And in memory of Darrin:
a life too short, a spirit never forgotten.

Contents

Acknowledgments

From the beginning of musing about what this book would be and how to communicate why empowerment is so essential to our good health, I knew one thing—I'd always approached health in a different way, and this book would be no exception. There are thousands of books out on any number of medical issues and conditions. Cures, theories, diets, you name it. But this was different. I didn't want to give one more opinion on what we are doing wrong when it comes to our health. I wanted to give readers the tools, the strength, and the insight to see that finding the power to take control of your health can be simple, can be done, and yes, can even be fun!

I've spent many years developing health programs, giving seminars, and talking with people about their health. I see how excited people get when they discover that they have the power to be healthier, to take charge and be more involved in their health. I wanted to somehow capture that excitement and bring it to life on the printed page. It was going to take the vision and dedication of lots of people to make this happen—people who could put aside their perceptions and embrace a new way to think about our health. So though the name on the front cover says "Taylor Grant," *Health Matters* is due to the efforts of a talented and dedicated group of people that transformed these ideas, experiences, and blank pages into the book that you now hold in your hands.

First, I thank my illustrating partner, Ann Sabo, for using her immense talents to bring my characters and stories to life. From her drawing of me (who came to be known as Tiggy) to my favorite— the

Ya-But "pixie"—Ann has an incredible knack for finding a unique take on a story. Her spirit, offbeat sense of humor, and pure talent made this not just a job, but a real labor of love and dedication.

I would especially like to thank all the folks at John Wiley & Sons, particularly my editor, Tom Miller, Juliet Grames, and everyone on the Wiley production staff. Tom, words aren't thanks enough for your vision in understanding the importance of empowering people to take control of their health and for your strength to look at health in an entirely new way. I thank Tom for his support, patience, and commitment. A big thank-you to Juliet Grames for her extraordinary attention to detail and for running interference for me, making my vision for this book come to life. To everyone on the production staff, I offer my gratitude for all your hard work maintaining the personality and integrity of the message. And to the marketing folks, your belief in the mission and reaching people with this message is a reflection of your dedication and professionalism.

I also want to thank my talented photographer, Dan Gaye, for turning a pumpkin into a princess! His infinite patience and determination to get me to smile—even after six hours—always amazes me.

You don't have to look far to find someone who will tell you how tough the world of publishing can be. I am fortunate enough to have the support and commitment of the best in the business—Dupree Miller & Associates. Jan Miller is a gracious, dedicated agent who defies cynics by believing that books cannot only change the world but can truly inspire people to change their lives. And I can't offer enough thanks to Nena Madonia for her seemingly endless supply of optimism, commitment, and talent for making a vision into a reality. This book would not have come to fruition without you in my corner. And to Michael Broussard, now at HarperCollins, thanks for pulling that envelope out of the stack and seeing the vision and for your no-holds-barred belief and encouragement.

I'd also like to thank Jillian Rowley, Health Editor at *Woman's Day* magazine, not to mention the *Woman's Day* readers whose overwhelming response gave me the determination to take this mission to the streets. Although she hardly knows it, it was Jillian who took a chance on an unknown author, seeing that sometimes the message matters more than the marketing.

Thank you also to Allan Rahn. Your support, encouragement, and never-faltering confidence have been an uplifting boost of "positivity" when it's needed the most. Thanks for the insight, thanks for the work, thanks for the good times, and thanks for being a true friend indeed.

I would be remiss not to thank my two "Bills" for always believing in the dream and always, always, working to make us look good. Bill Deering, you are a consummate professional, and I've never met a person with a better can-do attitude. Bill Hanson, it is truly just not the same without you. I still expect to see you when I walk through that door. I know you're somewhere watching, doing your crossword, and cheering on your beloved Sox.

To my mom and dad, thank you for instilling in me the powerful belief that I could do anything I set my mind to and for helping me to look at life's challenges with a sense of wonder and joy.

To my children, Sam and Jack, I have to say thanks for putting up with all the long hours, the trips around the country, and the endless talk about staying healthy. You make me laugh every single day, and I am in constant awe of the wonderful human beings you have become.

And most importantly, I have to thank my partner, my cheerleader, and my husband, John. First for setting aside his business interests to help me pursue this grandiose mission and reminding me every day that making a difference matters more than making a buck. Your knowledge and grasp of economics, free market demand, and statistical analysis helps keep my ideas and musings grounded in reality and made this book better than I could have hoped. Thank you for teaching me, more than anyone I've ever met, that taking a chance is what makes life worth living. I am always in awe of your ability to put it all on double zero, stand back, and watch that wheel spin. I thank you for your supreme confidence and unwillingness to let me ever give up.

And finally, thank you to everyone who has shared their health stories with me over the years. People love talking about their health and the health of their family, and I am so lucky because I love hearing their stories—it is my favorite part of what I do. I never cease to be amazed at the fortitude with which people address their challenges. And my belief in our strength, resiliency, and ability to embrace new ideas is reaffirmed on almost a daily basis. You may not see your name and you may not recognize your story, but it is you who have inspired every word.

Be well.

Taylor's First Law of Health

You are on your own.

Introduction

Who Put You in Charge?

An Ailing System

In my second year at the University of Tampa in Florida, I met Darrin Donahue. He was handsome, funny, and athletic. We had a class together and became study partners, and it was obvious that our friendship was heading toward something more. I was ending a three-year relationship with a steady boyfriend and Darrin was in a similar situation with his longtime girlfriend, so we decided just to be good friends, wrap things up with our exes, and take things slowly. We were in no hurry to rush into anything. We had all the time in the world.

Then one morning I got a call from my soon-to-be ex-boyfriend. "Darrin's dead," he said. I laughed nervously. It seemed that he'd figured out that Darrin and I were becoming more than friends. But that wasn't the case.

"I'm serious," he said. "Darrin collapsed in the shower this morning and he's dead. Well—he's in the hospital on life support until his eyes can be donated, but he's brain-dead. They found a brain tumor."

Just when I think I have learned the way to live, life changes.

—HUGH PRATHER, AUTHOR OF *SHINING THROUGH*

He reminded me then of how Darrin had always complained of headaches. His frat friends had chided him about being hungover, but he wasn't a big drinker. I'd even prodded him to go to the doctor, which he did, but the doctor told him it was nothing, so he'd laughed it off.

"You worry too much," he'd told me.

At Darrin's memorial service, I felt so guilty. Why hadn't I been more adamant about him going to the doctor? Why didn't any of us realize something was really wrong with him? He had symptoms—how could nobody know? Would he still be alive if he'd gotten some tests? I watched his parents and thought how their grief was simply unimaginable. A healthy, active, wonderful son. One day, off at college, playing on the tennis team, planning for his future. The next day, gone.

But most of all, I just felt an incredible sense of loss of what might have been for Darrin. He would never get the chance to graduate from college, never have a career, never get married and have kids. All his dreams, all his chances, gone in an instant.

I promised myself two things that day. First, I would make the most of every day—I would try to be happy and live life in the present, not wait until tomorrow. Second, I would always try to remember Darrin, to keep his memory alive—he deserved that. We didn't have a big relationship, had only known each other about a year, but somehow what made me the saddest was the life to come that Darrin and his family had lost. In my youthful naiveté I just didn't understand that this was a much more commonplace tragedy than I could have ever imagined and, inexplicably, would continue to become more and more common here, where we have the most respected health care system in the world.

Why I Do It

At one of the health seminars I hold around the country, someone once asked me why I do what I do. "Why do you care so much about health, why are you so passionate about it?" At first I didn't have a good answer. I mean, I'm not a doctor and never wanted to be one, though I grew up surrounded by them.

Although my mom and dad weren't doctors, I grew up in a medical family. My parents came from poor immigrant parents and were raised with a fierce work ethic that was passed along to my brother, sister, and me. My mother was the youngest of ten children whose father died when she was only ten years old. My father's mother—my grandmother—died from a minor infection when my dad was just four. Medicine was different then. Life was different then.

To my mom and dad, being a doctor was the highest achievement you could reach. They made many sacrifices to give their children the education and opportunities to achieve that goal. Both my brother and sister made it and today are practicing physicians.

Since I was the youngest, I grew up amidst a constant stream of medical jargon. Our Thanksgiving turkey was the only one in the neighborhood that was closed up with surgical sutures. But despite this, I never had the calling to be a doctor. Even as a youngster, when my brother or sister would take me to the hospital, I always felt more kinship with the patients than I did with the doctors. I was always fascinated by their stories, their point of view. I would pepper the doctors I met with questions about how they *felt* about their patients. Most of the time they would look at me strangely and talk about some surgical procedure they had planned for that day.

I was always intrigued by the way the doctors talked about the patients as "cases," rarely acknowledging that they were people. They never seemed interested in their families or their situations, just in curing them—and yet it was their stories, their lives, that fascinated me the most. Once I asked some brain surgery students how they felt about getting close to someone while knowing they might die. One young doctor told me, "I can't *get* close to them. My job is to save their lives. The only way I can do that is not to think of them as people with lives. That's just too hard. I've got a nine-year-old with a brain tumor. I can't get distracted thinking about how tragic it is. His family is counting on me to save his life."

I was blown away by the self-sacrifice and dedication of these doctors. But I also knew that I would never be able to give up that part of myself. Never be able to put those thoughts aside and see a person as just a "case." I knew that if I couldn't do that, I would be too emotionally involved to do the job I should for both my patients and myself.

So I went to work for the government, and after that, both corporations and nonprofit organizations, developing health, safety, and marketing programs to help people learn how to manage their health and their lives. And as I worked on these programs I became more and more aware of the disease that was infecting our health care system, making all of us sick, threatening our health, our safety, and our lives. I'm not the first or by any means the only person to note the dangerous direction our health care system is heading in, hurtling toward a real crisis. But instead of just sounding the alarm, I've become convinced that the only way we are possibly going to save this system and save ourselves would be if each of us took responsibility for our own health, start demanding the care and the life we each deserve, and begin to reform the system from the outside in.

As time went on, I became impassioned about turning the stories that people had told me about their health struggles into something positive that people could use to feel better and save their lives. I wanted to give people information, tools, and resources they could trust and use to help them make the decisions and choices that will let them live a healthy life, and a long one.

So one day I thought about it—about why I was doing it; about the course my life had taken that had brought me here, talking to you about your health. And I remembered Darrin.

You see, when you're healthy (and especially when you're young), your health doesn't seem to matter, and our health care system and how you interact with it seem like just a distant idea. The weird part is that when you're healthy you've got no reason to think about your health. You don't use the health care system—that's for *sick* people—so why worry about it?

But here's the thing: when you *do* need it, when that moment comes—you or someone you love gets sick or injured—you not only need it, you *rely* on it. It *must* be there and it *must* work well. Let's be honest. The system failed Darrin and his parents in the worst way it possibly could. And the thing is, it wasn't a fluke. It wasn't an accident. It wasn't just "one of those things." Darrin had symptoms. Darrin did what he was supposed to do—he went to the doctor. But when a strapping twenty-year-old walks into your office with a headache, it's easy to wave it off as nothing. Darrin didn't have to die like that. But it happens every day, hundreds if not thousands of times a day. It's happened to me. It's happened to people I love. It's happened to hundreds of people whom I've met who have told me their stories.

Missed conditions. Mixed-up medications. Treatments that don't work. Doctors who don't care. Test results that you aren't told about. People whose lives end way before they should. Families that lose children, mothers, fathers, grandfathers, brothers and sisters, aunts and uncles, and the love and joy that they bring to their lives. People who suffer through debilitating illnesses that could have been detected with a simple test.

I thought as I grew older that our health care system would get better. As we developed new medical discoveries and cures, people would stop dying. Well, I knew that people would still die, but I thought they wouldn't die because we didn't know they were sick. They wouldn't die because they got the wrong medicine or the wrong treatment or no treatment at all. They wouldn't die because we never thought to ask them how they felt. But the system kept evolving and people kept dying. In fact, the more time passed, the more people seemed to be dying unnecessarily. "Why?" I kept asking myself and everyone else. "When we've got the best medical system in the world?"

I got a thousand different answers, but none of them satisfied me. So I guess that's why I do it. Our system is sick. I know that I can't fix it on my own. But I can take what I've learned, take what I've heard, and turn it into something you can use to protect your life, keep you feeling better, and save the lives of those you love.

Did knowing Darrin lead me here? I don't know. I do know that I believe everything happens for a reason. I couldn't save Darrin's life. But maybe by having had the privilege to be Darrin's friend, maybe I can take that anger, that frustration, that sadness, and the sadness of everyone who's told me their stories, and use it to help others save their own lives or the life of someone they love. Because I've decided that even one more life, one more soul, lost because of mistakes, neglect, incompetence, or apathy is one life too many. Especially if it's yours.

The Coming Health Care Tsunami

I heard a story told by a ten-year-old British girl, Tilly Smith, shortly after she had witnessed the Indonesian tsunami in December 2004. Tilly was on vacation at the beach in Phuket, Thailand, with her family. She suddenly saw everyone staring at the tide, which was rushing out. They looked on in amazement because the water was quickly receding, rather than rolling in as it normally does. But this little girl had studied giant waves, called tsunamis, just two weeks before in her geography class and quickly realized they were in danger. She told her mother that they had to leave the beach immediately—which her mother passed on to the other people on the beach and at the hotel, more than a hundred people. Everyone quickly evacuated before the wave struck the beach minutes later. No one at the beach was seriously injured or killed.

I feel a little bit like Tilly. We're all standing at the beach—doctors, patients, the government, hospitals, drug companies, insurance companies, every one of us—looking at the water going out to sea, wondering, "Hmm? Why is it doing that?" That tide is our health care system. The water is rushing out to sea because a giant wave is building—a wave that's going to come crashing down on all of us, causing enormous amounts of harm. I'm not screaming "Run!" but I will tell you that if you don't get prepared, don't become more aware of your health and how to get the health care you need, that wave is going to come crashing over you and the people you love.

Let's take a look at a few figures that indicate some frightening trends in our health care system.

- **Dire shortage of family physicians predicted** The American Academy of Family Physicians is predicting a dire shortage of family physicians in at least five states and serious shortages in other states by the year 2020. The number of Americans needing more health care (because of aging and chronic conditions) is skyrocketing. The organization says that we'll need 40 percent more family doctors over the next fourteen years just to keep up with the demand. What's so disturbing is that not only are we *not* getting more doctors, the number of U.S. medical graduates going into family practice has *fallen* by over 50 percent from 1997 to 2005, as more young doctors choose to pursue specialty practices that offer better hours, higher pay, and more prestige.
- **Two-thirds of intensive care patients receive bad care** The Health and Human Services Department reported findings in May 2006 that two out of three patients who need critical care aren't getting proper care because of a serious shortage of critical care spe-

cialists (including doctors and nurses). This shortage results in the unnecessary deaths of up to 54,000 people every year.

- **Emergency care crisis** The Institutes of Medicine (a division of the National Academy of Sciences) issued a report in June 2006 on the frightening state of emergency medicine in the United States. On top of a critical shortage of emergency room and ICU doctors, emergency rooms are overcrowded, causing ambulances to be sent to other hospitals, delaying care. It's become common for emergency rooms to leave patients lying on gurneys or hospital beds parked in hallways (called boarding) for hours while they wait for someone to help them.
- **1.8 million people each year pick up infections in the hospital** These infections directly cause the death of 20,000 people each year and contribute to the death of 70,000 more. "But people have always gotten sick in the hospital—there's just more germs there," you might argue. But the rate of these infections has actually gone *up* 36 percent in the last twenty years, even as we've improved sterilization and developed drugs that fight infections. Health officials attribute this disturbing and deadly rise in infections to lax patient-safety practices in hospitals as well as the rise of antibiotic-resistant bacteria strains in response to an overuse of antibiotics.
- **One out of every five hundred people admitted to the hospital is killed by a mistake** Compare that to the chance of being killed in a commercial airline accident, which is one per eight million flights.
- **35 to 40 percent of missed diagnoses result in death** Prevention and early diagnosis isn't just a perk. It's what our system is supposed to be doing, yet it seems it's failing at an alarming rate.

So Who Put You in Charge

You'll notice that the heading for this section isn't phrased as a question, "Who Put You in Charge?," but rather as a statement. That's because there's no question about it: you are in charge. If you doubt that for a minute, let me tell you one person's story:

I was on a weekend cruise, relaxing for once, sitting on deck in the sun working at my computer (okay, only relaxing a little, but I was in the sun at least). A woman approached and asked if she could sit at my table and share my sunlight. "Please," I said, offering her a chair.

"You're just like my husband," she laughed, nodding her head to indicate her husband sitting at another table in the shade a few yards away, "always working. I can't believe you're here, looking at this beautiful ocean, and neither of you can shut off your computers and just relax."

Sensing she wanted to talk, I closed the lid of my laptop and snuggled into my chair for a nice chat. What I didn't expect was that I would still be working the way I usually do—listening to people's health stories.

"I'm trying to get my husband to slow down because he's been very sick."

"What has he been dealing with?" I asked.

"Pancreatic cancer. Very advanced, usually deadly. But he's out of the woods now, thank God. We had a tough battle, but it looks like he won."

Listening to the background of his condition and treatment, I became fascinated when she spoke about how they had gone about getting treatment. "We just decided to fight the fight of our lives. We weren't going to lie down and just watch him die. We used the Internet and books and friends and doctors to find out *everything* we could about the condition and what treatments were being used. We took charge of his condition [her words, not mine]. We found that there were only two doctors in the country that were doing the cutting-edge surgery that we thought he needed, so we refinanced our house and picked up and went to Texas to get the treatment. And we never gave up. We had bad days—lots of them. But we saw this as a battle for which the only acceptable outcome was victory and I'm just convinced that those two things—positive attitude and taking charge of our own care—are why my husband is sitting here today."

"That's amazing," I said. And I meant it. What a wonderful, uplifting story. I could just see the love that woman had for her husband and the appreciation she had for the gift of having him with her today. But I couldn't stop myself from thinking, "Why did it have to be that way? What about the people who didn't know they had to take matters into their own hands, seek out the right doctors, find the newest treatment; who gave up on themselves and died without having a fighting chance? Wasn't our system supposed to take care of them, too?"

As if reading my mind, the woman went on, "I know this is true because you'll never believe it. One year after my husband was diagnosed, our minister found out he had the very same type of cancer. We talked to him about it, about what we had found out, how we'd fought for our lives, but he just didn't want to hear it. You could see he had just given up. Six months later he died."

"I'm so sorry to hear that. That's a tragedy," I said.

"I still wish I could get my husband off that darned computer," she smiled.

The answer to who put you in charge is our health care system. Don't doubt for a minute the first of Taylor's Laws of Health that you'll see throughout this book: *you are on your own*.

You are on your own to make sure you don't suddenly get a life-threatening condition. You are on your own to make sure you don't have a bad reaction to a medication. You are on your own to keep yourself safe when you are in the hospital. And you are certainly on your own when you need the care that will save your life. But saying you're in charge and actually taking charge are two different things.

For some reason, when we enter the doctor's exam room, years of maturity, responsibility, and knowledge just get washed away and there we are, in that little paper gown, sitting on that cold exam table, feeling about eight years old. Not just physically naked, but emotionally naked as well. Afraid to say what we want. Intimidated that we just don't understand our own bodies. Embarrassed to talk about symptoms or admit to habits that are less than perfect. Our system was designed that way—to make us obedient patients who would listen to our doctors—but now that system has been turned on its head, putting your health, and your life, at risk.

The System Is Killing Us

Not only does the system do little to keep us from getting sick, in many instances it actually causes more problems than it fixes! Medical mistakes are a serious threat to your health and well-being. The total number of people who die every year from medical errors varies so widely and goes so unreported that I can't really state an exact figure here.

Take a look at some conservative estimates on medical mistakes:

Mistake	Estimated Deaths Every Year
Adverse drug reactions	106,000
Medical errors	98,000
Bedsores and infections	203,000
Unnecessary procedures	37,000

Add to this an estimate of 8.9 million unnecessary hospitalizations every year and it's enough to scare you into being healthy! In 1994, Dr. Lucien Leape published a paper in the *Journal of American Medicine* titled "Error in Medicine" that took a good, hard look at the harm our system was doing to our health. Dr. Leape compared the deaths from medical mistakes to the equivalent of *three jumbo jets crashing every two days*. At that error rate, I don't think any of us would ever get on a plane again. Leape also acknowledged that because the data on medical errors are sparse and since we know that the vast majority go unreported, his figures were probably very conservative. In fact, what Leape was saying is that a *lot* more people were dying than even his statistics, as troubling as they were, showed.

Leape hoped this report would "fundamentally change the way [the medical community thinks] about errors and why they occur." Sadly, over a decade later, no real changes have been made in our system, and people just keep dying. In fact, another report issued by the Institute of Medicine offered an even worse picture. In one part of their study, 1,047 patients admitted to a large teaching hospital were studied. Of those patients, 480, or *46 percent*, had an adverse event—a situation where a bad decision was made. For 185 of those patients, the adverse event was serious, causing disability or death. Do the math on the number of patients in every hospital in the United States and the figure is astounding.

How could it be that a system that's supposed to *save* our lives instead *kills* more people each year than all other accidents combined? That hospitals are literally more dangerous than war zones? To understand why these mistakes continue to happen, you have to understand how our medical system works.

Nobody's Perfect, Right?

Our medical system operates on an infallibility model. It's assumed that the doctors, nurses, technicians, and other people who provide your care will never make a mistake—will be infallible. "What's so wrong with that?" you might ask. Well, for starters, you and I both know (and the system seems to demonstrate) that none of us is infallible. We all make mistakes. But having a system where perfection is presumed means that each person down the line assumes that what the person before them did was correct and so does nothing to double-check, take any steps to catch an error, or correct any errors that could have occurred, because, according to the system, no errors ever occur. This means that often errors get worse and worse and worse as they are compounded all down the line, eventually, in the worst cases, resulting in a patient's death.

Even worse, there is such a stigma against reporting errors that almost all mistakes are swept under the carpet. This means they're never examined to see how they could be prevented from happening again. It's estimated that only 1.5 percent of all mistakes are ever reported, mostly by patients themselves! Doctors and nurses, living in fear of malpractice suits and disciplinary actions, have no training and no motivation to prevent and fix mistakes.

Doctors are suffering at the hands of our system as well. More and more medical students are being forced to turn away from what they love—treating patients—and turn to more lucrative specialties like plastic surgery, dermatology, and eye surgery.

A doctor whose daughter was in the same kindergarten class as my daughter told me of his struggle.

> I'm a family practice doctor—it's what I like to do—but I'm going to have to give it up. I feel like I've tried everything but nothing's working. First I took a job with a big medical practice as one of their staff physicians. But I was just asked to grind out as many appointments a day as possible—get 'em in, get 'em out, I used to say—and it just didn't feel like I could give people the care I wanted to. So I decided to open my own practice. I could see from the medical group that there sure wasn't a lack of patients. But soon after I got started, I could see there was going to be a problem. I signed on with some health insurance

> plans and even some government plans. I agreed to take Medicare patients because I have a lot of experience with senior care. I started seeing patients and at first it was great. I took my time, went over their history, ordered tests and screenings. Then I started filing my claims. Oh my gosh. I admit it, the business side of being a doctor has never been my thing. I mean, I can do it, but I like concentrating on the patients. But anyway, the reimbursement rates were so low that I couldn't even pay my office rent every month. One government plan paid me ten dollars for an office visit. These office visits were taking me around thirty minutes each. So I started doing what I was doing before, trying to move patients in and out as quickly as possible. But that's just frustrating to both them and me. I know I need to be efficient, but I just don't think I can give people the care I think they need under these circumstances. I'm going to start making mistakes and missing things and I just don't want to practice like that.

That's why it's so important for *you* to be on top of your health and take charge of your care every step of the way. You are your own best advocate, and many times you are your only advocate. Even the most dedicated, talented doctors make mistakes and feel the push to move faster, do more. It's your job, your responsibility, to do everything you can to help them do their job right to protect your life.

But as you set out to take charge of your health, one of the challenges you face is how to sort through all of the information, the mixed messages, and the onslaught of marketing that are thrown at you about your health every single day.

Headline Health

Take a look at these headlines, taken from a single day's news.

> HOW CLEAN IS THE ICE IN YOUR DRINK?
>
> LOW-FAT DIET SAVES LIVES!
>
> SCIENTISTS WARN OF ANIMAL-DISEASE RISK
>
> LOW-FAT DIET A BUST
>
> ESTROGEN TIED TO STROKE RISK

And these are just the reputable ones. I'm not trying to pick on the news media. Hidden in these screaming headlines is some great information about your health. But what's a person to do? Eat low-fat. Don't eat low-fat. Carbs are bad. Carbs are good. Take this drug. No, wait! It might kill you.

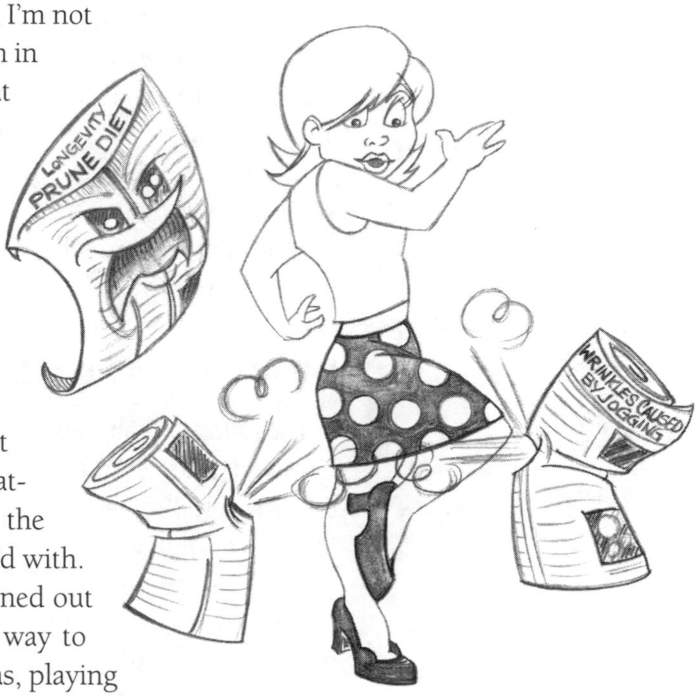

Nobody's counting, but I'd estimate that the average American sees or hears over twenty health stories a day. It's what I call *headline health*. Without someone to guide and advise you, it's natural to try to take what you can from the information that you're constantly blasted with. But consumers are just getting plain burned out on headline health, and frankly, it's no way to run a health care system. Michael Douglas, playing the title role in *The American President*, said, "In the absence of genuine leadership, people will listen to anyone who steps up to the microphone. They want leadership. They're so thirsty for it they'll crawl through the desert toward a mirage, and when they discover there's no water, they'll drink the sand."

I think that's the way most of us feel about our health. We know we need to take care of our health. We know it's important—what we eat, how much we weigh, if we get the right tests. The thing is, there's no one out there telling us how to do that. We aren't taught about it in school. Our doctors aren't really doing it. The government issues as many confusing statements as the next guy, so we're taking our direction where we can get it—from the headlines. In effect, we're drinking the sand.

It is my hope that this book can help you find a way through all of that. Once you've embraced the fact that you and you alone are in charge of your health and that you can make choices and take actions that affect how long you live and the quality of your life, I know you'll find the strength to take on that challenge.

As I travel around the country, I am awed by the knowledge, motivation, and strength people demonstrate about their health. Like that woman on the cruise, people tell me stories of finding new treatments when nothing seemed to work, finding the determination to beat illnesses and manage conditions so they can lead full, happy lives. It's incredibly inspiring to hear those stories and see how people are working and fighting to get all they can out of life.

So I hope I've answered the people who have asked me, "Why does it matter so much to you?" and I hope you understand why it has to matter so much to *you*.

Let's Get This Party Started

In the following chapters, you'll find 8 Prescriptions for Life that will help you understand why we avoid dealing with our health. You'll discover what's essential to understanding your body and your health. I'll tell you how you can harness your Health Power to get good medical care, make positive changes in your life, and do what's needed to protect your family. You'll find these pages packed with useful tools, including evaluations to help you look at what motivates you as well as forms and checklists that will help you organize your health and understand exactly what you need to do. You'll also find lots of unusual health facts I call Know Way!, along with Pop Quizzes to test your knowledge about your body and your health. My 5-Minute Clinics will give you quick tips you can use to protect yourself and stay healthy. Each prescription also comes loaded with resources such as Web sites and books you can use to get more information, find great doctors, or even give your memory a workout.

You'll also read stories of people who, just like you and me, have struggled with their health, done battle in the health care system, and, many times, come out victorious. As a small note about those stories, with few exceptions, the names, identifying details, and even circumstances about the people I write about have been changed. While I believe that no health issue is anything to be ashamed of or embarrassed about, I also know that your health information is the most personal information you have, and I respect the privacy of those who have been kind enough to relate their stories to me.

So if someday we ever meet (and I hope we do), please tell me your *healthstory*. I love to hear them! And while I might use what you've accomplished to help others, your privacy will always be sacred.

So let's get started taking these eight prescriptions and put them to work to give you the longest, healthiest, happiest life possible.

Before you dive into Prescription 1, I'd like you to do a small warm-up exercise.

Life Priorities Audit

This Life Priorities Audit will help you think about how you view your health in relation to the other aspects of your life. It's going to help you see where you place your feelings about your health in five life aspects: control, motivation, priorities, relationships, and spirituality.

There's no right or wrong answers to this audit. Remember, it's all about *you* and how you feel about your health. This audit will help you answer other questions as you move through the 8 Prescriptions as well as evaluate your progress as you begin to feel more in control.

Life Priorities Audit

Control

Which aspect of your health are you most in control of?

____

____

Which aspect of your health are you least in control of?

____

____

Motivation

Which part of your life gives you the most satisfaction?

____

____

Which part of your life would you most like to change?

____

____

(continued)

Life Priorities Audit (continued)

Priorities

List your top five priorities in life (consider where you place your health).

1. ______________________________
2. ______________________________
3. ______________________________
4. ______________________________
5. ______________________________

Relationships

Which two people have the greatest influence on your health?

____

____

Which two people do you rely on most for help and support?

____

____

Which two people most depend on you for health support?

____

____

Spirituality

List the five things you do for your mind and body that give you the greatest sense of joy and tranquillity.

1. ______________________________
2. ______________________________
3. ______________________________
4. ______________________________
5. ______________________________

List the five things you do to your mind and body that are the most harmful to your physical and emotional well-being.

1. ______________________________
2. ______________________________
3. ______________________________
4. ______________________________
5. ______________________________

Taylor's Second Law of Health

Treat your health as your most valuable asset. It is.

Prescription 1

Conquer Your Fears

The Beginning of the End

Many books show you how to begin something: a diet, a business, a financial plan. This book is about ending something: ending a passive approach to your most valuable asset—your health; ending the frustration you feel when dealing with doctors or anyone in our health care system; ending the fear that somewhere inside a disease is lurking, waiting to claim your well-being, your peace of mind, or your life, and you are powerless against it.

By picking up this book, you've made a life-changing decision. You've realized that your health is too important to leave up to somebody else. You know that in order to live the longest life you can, you've got to understand your own health, have a plan to protect yourself, and take charge of your health and your life.

The National Center for Educational Statistics says that five out of six people have only *intermediate* health literacy skills—the ability to understand health information and use that information to make decisions about our health and our life. Their study shows that very few of us are proficient when it comes to understanding our health. And these results don't seem to have much to do with our reading literacy or educational levels. We're all stumped. The health information we're given is too technical and filled with too much jargon. For example, to help us eat less salt, we have to scour the ingredients list on a can of green beans to find the *sodium content*. While we hear story after story filled with health scares, warnings, and advice, we have virtually no training, experience, or help on how all of this information can be used in our own lives to make us feel better and stay healthy. It's this ignorance that keeps us from doing what we should to be healthier and traps us in the darkness of fear about our health rather than the power of enlightenment.

What Are the Odds?

Mad cow disease:
1 in 40 million

Shark attack:
1 in 10 million

Struck by lightning:
1 in 576,000

Finding a four-leaf clover:
1 in 10,000

Having a shaving injury:
1 in 6,600

Catching a baseball at major league game:
1 in 563

Having a stroke:
1 in 6

Developing diabetes:
1 in 3

Dave, a man who successfully battled cancer, described to me the effect this ignorance, early in his diagnosis and treatment, had on both his body and his mind:

> The worst part, truly the worst—more than the nausea, losing my hair, fearing death—was not knowing, not understanding what was happening to me. Each time the doctor ordered a test or treatment, I'd spend the night before with cold sweats, dreading not only the procedure itself, but even getting the results. And most of the time I didn't even know why I was having the test at all. Once I decided to stop being ignorant and get information so I could understand everything that was happening to me—*before* it happened—most of my fear just evaporated. Just knowing, understanding, asking questions and getting answers, empowered me in a way I never thought was possible. I felt better, more in control. I'm convinced it's what made me get better. That fear of the unknown was eating at me, almost making me feel like just letting the cancer win.

Face Your Fears

Everyone has fears about their health—we just don't talk about them very often. Like all fears, they make us uncomfortable. They come from the dark recesses of our childhood and touch on topics that get at our very core: pain, suffering, loss of control, loss of loved ones, death.

It's normal to feel uncomfortable talking about a health condition with someone who's battling an illness. What do you say? What's too personal? How do you show you really care and want to help? Thankfully, we've moved away from the days when we would discuss someone's condition with whispers and nods. But while we talk about the treatments and the trips to the doctor, we still tiptoe around the subject of our fears and our feelings. The Health Fears Appraisal, beginning on page 20, will help you examine your health fears in five key areas: your health, your family, your work, your health care team, and your financial matters. Answer these questions honestly to help you understand where your fears may be holding you back from living your healthiest, longest life.

> To conquer fear is the beginning of wisdom.
>
> —BERTRAND RUSSELL, PHILOSOPHER

I'm going to help you put an end to the fears and behaviors that keep you from feeling your best and may even shorten your life. You'll learn to pull back the shutters on your fears, bring them out into the light, and separate what's irrational from what's real. I'll give you simple steps you can take to be in control of your health. And most importantly, you'll start breaking those bonds of ignorance, taking off the blinders, and finding the power to become an expert on your own health. Together, we'll examine feelings about

- fears about your health matters
- your health power and perceptions
- your doctors
- your family's health
- your commitment to a healthy life

You'll learn how to harness the positive power of those feelings to build a real-life plan you can use to begin your journey toward health, wellness, and happiness.

The Monster in Your Closet

Ignoring your health doesn't mean that you don't think about it. As you probably learned when you scored your Health Fears Appraisal, we have a complicated relationship with our health. In many ways we obsess about it—there are thousands of health stories every day on the Internet, in the newspaper, and on television. Drugstore shelves are packed with remedies, cures, vitamins, and medicines. We talk

Health Fears Appraisal

Health Matters	Disagree	⟷		Agree
1. If I couldn't do things that I enjoy (for example, sports, travel, reading), due to illness, I would be miserable.	1	2	3	4
2. I'm afraid that if I get sick, I will be ignored and avoided by other people.	1	2	3	4
3. If I were to get sick, I would be embarrassed to tell others about my condition or to ask for help in coping with my condition.	1	2	3	4
4. I am scared to face the truth about my health because I fear it will be bad news.	1	2	3	4
5. I don't want to think about the prospect that someday I will die.	1	2	3	4
6. I worry that getting sick could affect my ability to have sex.	1	2	3	4

Scoring and Evaluation

My Score ____________________

Evaluation

21–24 You're letting your fears get in the way of your good health. Instead, take control of your health with prevention and healthier choices.

16–20 While some fears are reasonable, they may be keeping you from living your healthiest life. Embrace your health and take charge to feel great!

11–15 Make a little more effort to face your fears head-on to put yourself at ease.

6–10 Keep building on your strengths to stay in control of your health.

FEAR ALERT

Confronting your health situation need not be scary. With a little effort, you can take charge of your health and feel at ease. Start by taking the Personal Health Assessment, then develop your Healthy Life Plan. Use these as a starting point to take control of your health.

Health Fears Appraisal

Family Matters	Disagree ⟷ Agree			
1. I don't have family members whom I can rely on if I have health problems.	1	2	3	4
2. I worry that I will be a burden to my family if I have an illness that I can't handle myself.	1	2	3	4
3. I don't think I am strong enough to handle the situation if a member of my family or another loved one gets sick and/or requires long-term care.	1	2	3	4
4. I have too many members of my family relying on me for me to get sick.	1	2	3	4
5. I am afraid that I might have inherited or passed along health conditions within my family.	1	2	3	4
6. I worry that I don't do enough to protect the health of my family or encourage healthy habits.	1	2	3	4

Scoring and Evaluation

My Score ____________________

Evaluation

21–24 Unfortunately, you're too old to be adopted! Try to bring your family together, strengthen your support network, and develop healthy lifestyles.

16–20 Work on improving your support system. Consider widening your circle to include friends, coworkers, and others.

11–15 Look for ways to improve your family's health and support.

6–10 You have a great family support system. Are you willing to adopt others?

FEAR ALERT

Relationships with your family and friends are one of your greatest health assets, so keep them strong. Your family health history is also an important legacy. It's not just genetics you inherit or pass on, but healthy (or not so healthy) habits like eating, exercise, stress management, and so on.

(continued)

Health Fears Appraisal (continued)

Work Matters	Disagree ⟷ Agree			
1. If I were to get sick, I would have difficulty keeping my current job or finding another one.	1	2	3	4
2. My employer is not concerned about my health, and my work environment is not safe or health-friendly.	1	2	3	4
3. I don't feel comfortable discussing concerns about my health with my employer because I think they will judge me or treat me differently.	1	2	3	4
4. I worry that I won't be paid if I miss work because of illness, and this would be a financial hardship.	1	2	3	4
5. I am concerned that my employer does not provide adequate health coverage for my family's needs.	1	2	3	4
6. I would be embarrassed if my coworkers found out that I had a health condition.	1	2	3	4

Scoring and Evaluation

My Score ________________

Evaluation

21–24 Your work environment creates a lot of stress about your health. Develop contingency plans and do more on your own to protect your health.

16–20 Your work environment needs some work. Make sure you explore all the options available both through work and on your own.

11–15 You may need to do some research and make efforts on your own to stay healthy and shore up your situation.

6–10 You have a health-friendly work environment. Keep up the good job!

FEAR ALERT Working in an environment that doesn't promote wellness can be hazardous to your health. There's a lot more to employee health than workplace safety. Talk to your employer about what they're doing to help you stay well.

Health Fears Appraisal

Health Care Team Matters	Disagree ⟵			⟶ Agree
1. I'm afraid to go to the doctor because I'm afraid I will get bad news.	1	2	3	4
2. I am embarrassed to talk with my doctor about problems with my body.	1	2	3	4
3. I am afraid that not having a doctor who manages and cares about my health may be putting my life and my health at risk.	1	2	3	4
4. I don't like to talk with my doctor because he or she will think I'm stupid.	1	2	3	4
5. I believe my doctor cares more about making money than about taking care of my health.	1	2	3	4
6. I am afraid to go into the hospital for fear that I will never come out.	1	2	3	4

Scoring and Evaluation

My Score ____________________

Evaluation

21–24 Strike out! Your relationship with your team is not healthy. Having doctors you trust and can work with is crucial to your health and well-being.

16–20 Pop fly! You need to get off the bench and scout some new doctors.

11–15 Base hit! Examine how you can improve your relationship with your doctors and find doctors who care about you to play on your team.

6–10 Home run! You're working well together, but don't stop there. Look for ways to make sure you're doing all you can on your end to be healthy.

FEAR ALERT Your health care team should have all your bases covered. If you're not happy with one of your team members, don't hesitate to make a trade. By the same token, a team is only as good as its manager (you). So get in there and play ball.

(continued)

Health Fears Appraisal (continued)

Financial Matters	Disagree ⟵⟶ Agree			
1. I can't afford to get sick because I won't be able to work and pay my bills.	1	2	3	4
2. If I get sick, I worry that I will lose my health insurance or be unable to get coverage.	1	2	3	4
3. I worry that I am damaging my health by avoiding treatments or drugs because I can't afford them.	1	2	3	4
4. If I have major medical bills, I am afraid that I won't be able to pay them and may have to declare bankruptcy.	1	2	3	4
5. I worry that I cannot afford a medical emergency for a member of my family.	1	2	3	4
6. I believe I would put my family at risk of losing our way of life if I were to get sick.	1	2	3	4

Scoring and Evaluation

My Score ____________________

Evaluation

21–24 You need outside help or advice to help you get the care you need and establish a medical safety net.

16–20 Develop a plan to avoid financial hardship—insurance, aid, new job, and so on.

11–15 Look for ways to strengthen your medical financial situation.

6–10 Even people with health insurance can get hit with big medical expenses. Make sure you've covered all your bases and get good preventive care.

Most personal bankruptcies in the United States are related to becoming ill. If you are uninsured, look into programs that your state and local government offer. Don't wait until an emergency arises to get the information you need!

about our health, think about it, and fret about it. But at the same time, in many important ways, we neglect it, figuring we'll do something about it tomorrow.

I like to call our health the monster hiding in the closet. You know it's there, but as long as you don't open the door, you'll be okay, right? You get up, you go to work, and you feel okay. That monster's asleep in the closet and everything's fine. But then . . . you feel a lump in your breast . . . you wake up on the floor and can't remember how you got there . . . you see blood where blood shouldn't be. That monster's awake now, and he's a bigger beast than you ever imagined. You're scared.

Shutting that monster in the closet isn't just a bad plan, it's a deadly one. But too often, it's the way we deal with our health. Why, when we know the monster's in there? We're too busy, too distracted, or have better ways to use our time—and often it's because that little monster can be pretty darn scary.

In this age of sometimes excruciating self-exploration and self-revelation, celebrities and just regular Joes alike line up on Oprah, Dr. Phil, Larry King, and—heaven help us—Howard Stern to reveal their deepest, darkest secrets. We talk about everything—it seems nothing is off-limits anymore. Facing Your Inner Child; Overcoming Your Fear of Success; I'm Okay, How Come You're Not?—we're willing to look our inner selves in the mirror and say, "Ha! Fear doesn't live here anymore!" Except, it seems, when it comes to our health. It's one of the last fears we seem reluctant to conquer. Why is health something most of us just want to avoid?

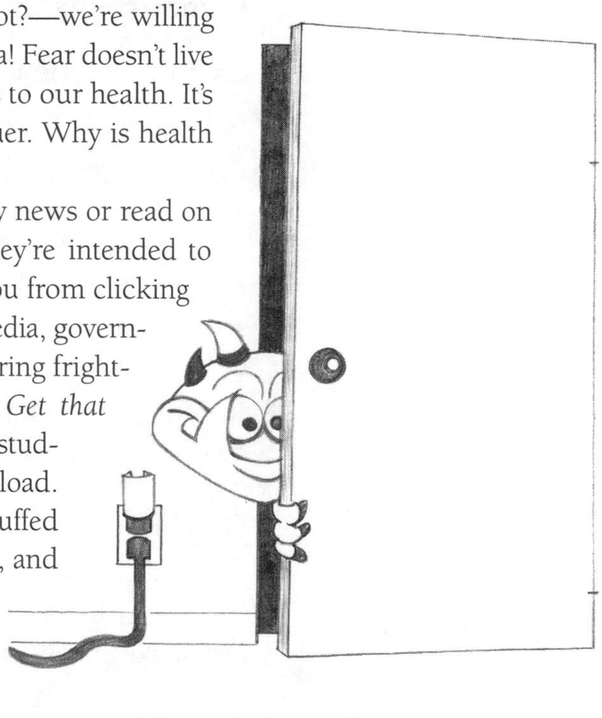

The health headlines you hear on the nightly news or read on the Internet can be downright frightening. They're intended to scare you into listening or reading (and keep you from clicking off to somewhere else). And many folks in the media, government, and our health care system think that hearing frightening statistics might scare you into action. *Get that prostate exam or die!* They mean well, but in fact, studies have shown that most people are on overload. Daily reports on health risks and scares have stuffed our closets full of monsters in every size, shape, and color, and we've decided it's easier to just slam that door shut than figure out what to do. Vague threats are announced without specifics to help us understand who is at risk and how real a threat is. Take breast cancer, for example. You don't often hear it reported that 70 percent of women who get it don't die from it. And if women took advantage of early screenings and treatment, more than 95 percent could survive. Elaine Ratner, author of *The Feisty Woman's Breast Cancer Book*, says that the publicity given to breast cancer in an effort to drive women toward prevention and detection has created a false impression that breast cancer is far more common than it is. Ratner believes that this fear has actually had the opposite effect, making women avoid tests and examinations that could save their lives.

RESOURCE

Health Myths for Women

Get the facts on common health myths for women at www.cdc.gov/women/owh/myths.

Jessie Gruman, president of the Center for Advancement of Health, says that the media plays a big part in stoking these fears. "The problem is that mass media fly on news, meaning information has to be tarted up to be used. This plants the seeds of fear instead of education."

But health scares are not reserved just for today's twenty-four-hour cable news channels. America has a rich heritage of hysteria and hype when it comes to health. Let's take a look at some infamous health scares of our past and present.

Famous Health Scares in History

Lethal Tomatoes

Scare April 1812: Tomatoes are poisonous and will kill you.

Fact Although Italians had been growing and eating tomatoes since 1550, Americans didn't start eating them until around 1830 because they were widely thought to be poisonous. Legend has it that Colonel Robert Gibbon Johnson introduced the tomato to Salem, Massachusetts, by publicly eating a basket of tomatoes in the town square. He drew quite a crowd of gawkers, who expected to watch him die.

Result Can you imagine food without tomatoes? Pizza Hut might be called Flat Bread Cheese Shack.

Don't Pass the Cranberry Sauce

Scare November 1959: U.S. Secretary of Health, Education, and Welfare Arthur Fleming announced that a shipment of cranberries examined in San Francisco had traces of aminotriazole, a pesticide that hadn't yet been evaluated by the government but hadn't shown any danger. He casually warned, just fifteen days before Thanksgiving, that to be safe Americans probably shouldn't buy cranberries at all until the chemical could be tested further.

Fact The pesticide affected only a small portion of the total U.S. crop and wasn't found to be dangerous. For a person to ingest the same amount of the chemical that lab animals received in testing, he would have to eat 15,000 pounds of cranberries every day for years.

Result Secretary Fleming's offhand comment caused a panic about cranberries. The risk to humans from consuming cranberries was infinitesimal. On the campaign trail for the 1960 presidential election, Vice President Richard Nixon and Senator John Kennedy both consumed cranberries to show Americans that there was no danger.

Swine Flu Is Coming

Scare March 1976: A soldier at Fort Dix in New Jersey died from the "killer flu." Americans were whipped into a frenzy by reports that an epidemic was about to hit the United States. President Ford authorized a $135 million immunization program, and about 40 million Americans received shots.

Fact The soldier was the only person to die from the virus, and no epidemic developed. In a tragic irony, the vaccine itself caused an adverse reaction in some people, sickening hundreds and killing twenty-five—more than the disease itself.

Result This is probably the biggest overreaction to a health scare in our history and highlighted the power of the modern media to generate health hysteria. What's referred to by many health experts as the "Swine Flu Fiasco" is said to have diminished Americans' faith in health pronouncements from the government and rocked our confidence in the government to respond prudently to a potential large-scale contagious outbreak.

Coffee Causes Cancer

Scare February 1981: A study claimed that drinking two cups of coffee per day doubles your chances of getting pancreatic cancer, while drinking five cups per day triples your risk.

Fact The flawed study was published by a Harvard doctor whose findings could never be reproduced. There has not been any evidence since to suggest that coffee causes cancer.

Result Unbelievably, coffee sales were not affected by the study. This illustrates the danger that can come from putting too much emphasis on the results of a single study.

Can You Heal Me Now? Cell Phones and Brain Tumors

Scare 1990: An urban legend circulated and was picked up by the media that magnetic fields produced by a cell phone will cause brain tumors.

Fact While it is not possible to prove that electromagnetic fields (EMF) are safe, they have never been clearly linked with cancer.

Result Incidence of brain tumors has risen slightly in recent years, but not in proportion with the increase of cell phone use. The real danger of cell phones is using them while driving. Drivers using cell phones are four times as likely to have an accident as nonusers.

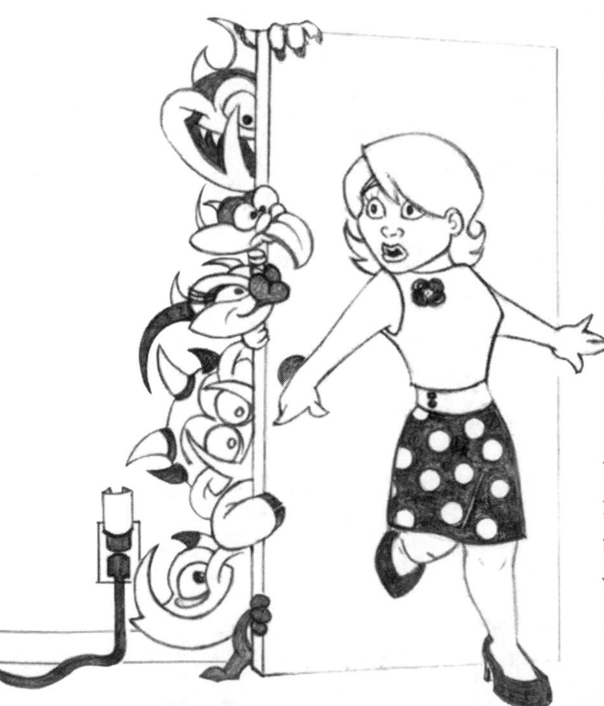

Bird Flu Pandemic

Scare Summer 2005: Fear spread that a lethal strain of flu would migrate from birds (no pun intended) to humans, causing a worldwide pandemic and killing millions of people.

Fact Common flu strains often go from birds to humans and are not necessarily life-threatening. The most recent bird flu strain causing concern, H5N1, has been linked to the deaths of slightly over a hundred people who came into direct contact with poultry, primarily in Asian and Eastern European countries. While scientists are concerned that the virus may gain the rare ability to be transmitted from human to human, which *might* cause a widespread flu epidemic, there is currently no evidence that this has occurred.

Result Being prepared for an epidemic of any kind is a challenge for the health care system in every country. The difficulty comes in deciding how much money and resources to direct toward a health problem that in all probability will never materialize, when at the same time millions of people aren't being treated for conditions like heart disease, diabetes, and asthma—conditions that are killing people every day.

You vs. the Monster

With all the scary news that you are bombarded with every day, battling the monster in your closet can be hard, partly because some health fears do contain a kernel of truth. No one can promise you that you won't get cancer or that you'll never have a heart attack. Your doctor can't guarantee "Disease-free or your money back!"

What's Your Real Risk?

What's interesting is that many of the things that seem to get the most press and invade our thoughts are things that, statistically, we have a very low risk of falling victim to (such as a terrorist attack, a plane crash, an epidemic). By contrast, some of the health issues that should get our attention (including heart disease, stroke, diabetes, and car accidents) don't seem to generate as much fear and, as a result, not much action to prevent and treat.

The Health Fear or Health Fiction checklist will help you evaluate whether a risk is something you should take seriously or one that just merits some interested watching. On page 30, you can see a sample I've done for a current health threat—bird flu—that's getting lots of news coverage. Be sure to evaluate the actual threat, not the "what if" scenario that usually gets the most attention. For example, you might say, "Hey, isn't the bird flu

Health Fear or Health Fiction

Should I Be Worried?

Use the following guide to help evaluate if you should be worried about the latest health scare.

1.	Did the information come from a credible source?	**Yes**	No
2.	Is it contagious?	**Yes**	No
3.	Is it easily transmitted or acquired?	**Yes**	No
4.	Is there an available vaccine?	Yes	**No**
5.	Is there an available treatment?	Yes	**No**
6.	Can you avoid the source (for example, airborne viruses as opposed to a particular contaminated food)?	Yes	**No**
7.	Is it in your geographic area?	**Yes**	No
8	Are you in a high-risk group?	**Yes**	No
9.	Does it have a serious or even deadly effect?	**Yes**	No
10.	Has it affected a large number of people?	**Yes**	No

Scoring and Evaluation

(Count the bold responses you circled.)

My Score __________

Evaluation

8–10 Take it seriously.

5–7 Take precautions but don't panic.

0–4 Just pay attention to it.

Sample Health Care Evaluation: Bird Flu

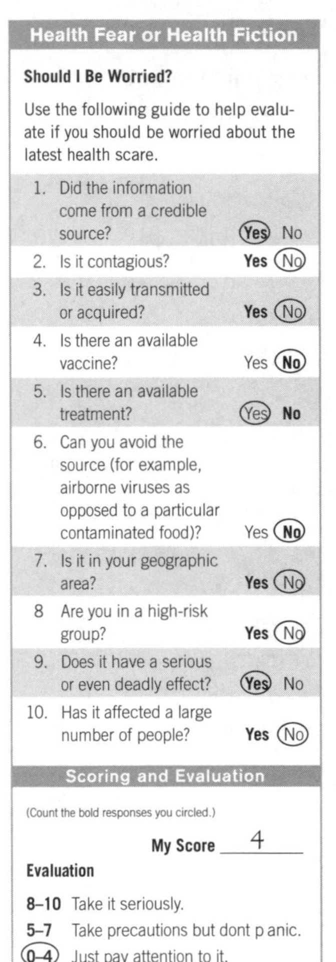

Health Fear or Health Fiction

Should I Be Worried?

Use the following guide to help evaluate if you should be worried about the latest health scare.

1.	Did the information come from a credible source?	(**Yes**) No
2.	Is it contagious?	**Yes** (No)
3.	Is it easily transmitted or acquired?	**Yes** (No)
4.	Is there an available vaccine?	Yes (**No**)
5.	Is there an available treatment?	(Yes) **No**
6.	Can you avoid the source (for example, airborne viruses as opposed to a particular contaminated food)?	Yes (**No**)
7.	Is it in your geographic area?	**Yes** (No)
8	Are you in a high-risk group?	**Yes** (No)
9.	Does it have a serious or even deadly effect?	(**Yes**) No
10.	Has it affected a large number of people?	**Yes** (No)

Scoring and Evaluation

(Count the bold responses you circled.)

My Score 4

Evaluation

8–10 Take it seriously.
5–7 Take precautions but dont p anic.
(**0–4**) Just pay attention to it.

contagious—why did you answer 'no' to number two?" The fact is that as of this writing, the bird flu has been transmitted only from bird to human (and even then on a very limited basis) and not from human to human. Every threat in the world has the potential to morph into something deadly; what you want to evaluate is the actual threat to you today. You can even use this list for conditions like diabetes and heart disease. While it is just a general guide, it can help you decide when your worries are worthy and when it's better to watch and wait.

How to Cope with Your Fears

The following strategies will help you from getting overwhelmed with negative headlines and information overload and will keep things in perspective.

- **Don't go it alone.** Being alone can isolate you and let you be overcome with your fears. Getting out and being around other people will remind you of the simple pleasures of life and help you get another view on the issues.
- **Ask for help if you need it.** If you're truly worried and need help coping, talk to your doctor, a family member, a social worker, or a friend. You may not realize that your fears have turned into an anxiety issue or panic attacks. Talking to someone will also help you understand the real risks and get help doing what you can to minimize those.
- **Help other people.** Many people who have lived through traumatic experiences or disasters report that it was saving other people that helped them get through the disaster and forget about their own problems. Thinking about those who need help will take the focus off yourself.
- **Understand that sometimes life is random.** Even people who take every precaution, live the healthiest life, and do everything right can have an accident or get sick, while people who smoke, drink, and hang-glide can live to be ninety. It's impossible to eliminate every danger in life, and you probably wouldn't want to even if you could. All you can do is try to take reasonable steps to reduce your risks and live the healthiest, safest life you can while still doing the things you love.

- **Enjoy your life.** Letting your fear overtake you is just giving in to a negative outlook. If you let fear keep you from doing what you should to be healthy or live a good life, you're letting the fear win. Time is too precious to throw away on being afraid.

When Fear Interferes

If you suspect your health fears have gotten out of hand, ask yourself the following questions to determine if you are coping with your fears or if they are overwhelming your life. Answering "yes" to one or more of the questions below may mean you should talk to a doctor, counselor, family member, or friend to make sure you aren't getting paralyzed by your fears.

- Are you worried or anxious most of the time?
- Do you feel hopeless about your future?
- Do your health fears make you avoid doctor appointments, get preventive care, or manage your health conditions?

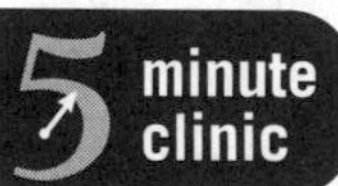

6 Ways to Keep Your Health Fears in Check

1. **Turn off the TV.** News channels tend to cover the same stories during the day, often giving a false sense of importance to minor issues. Wait a few days and see if the story continues to get coverage or if it was just the "press release of the day."
2. **Call your doctor if you're worried.** Don't call in a panic at 3 A.M., but it's fine to call during normal business hours and ask if there's anything to be concerned about.
3. **Don't start stockpiling the latest hyped-up cure.** Not only does this add to the mania, but it will almost certainly waste your money and time and might even be dangerous.
4. **Get the facts.** It can be hard to find reliable information amidst all the hysteria. Look for articles or Internet sites authored by reputable, unbiased sources. The *Daily Tattler* may not be your best source of health information despite their crack reporting on two-headed alien babies.
5. **Consider your actual odds.** Put your risk in perspective. Your odds of encountering anthrax are about a zillion to one (not a real statistic).Your odds of getting injured in an automobile accident are 1 in 75. The risk of an accident doesn't stop you from getting into your car—you just try to drive safely. Well, some people do. Not the people where I drive, but some people. Don't let the media-reported "risks" keep you from living your life.
6. **Take positive action where it counts.** Being afraid without doing anything is just wasting your emotions. For example, if you are afraid of catching the flu, washing your hands more often is a simple thing you can do to reduce your risk and, hopefully, your fear.

RESOURCE

Check Out Product Safety and Recalls

Get the latest on product recalls at 800-638-2772 or click on www.cpsc.gov.

- Do you have trouble sleeping?
- Do your health fears keep you from traveling, socializing, or doing other activities that make you happy?
- Do you feel isolated and alone?
- Does your worrying interfere with your work or personal relationships?
- Do you use drugs or alcohol excessively to cope with your feelings of anxiety?

It's also important to remember that worrying about your health is completely normal and, in fact, isn't always bad. If you keep it in perspective and don't let it overpower you, fear, in small doses, can help motivate you to make positive changes in your life. Fear can make you look for a better job, plan for your retirement, or adopt new habits. But too often, fears about your health have just the opposite effect. Since we aren't sure what to do to manage our own health, we would just rather avoid the subject altogether. Keep the monster in the closet where he belongs. Take me, for example.

I recently went to the doctor for a condition that had been bothering me. Nothing serious, just something that was sort of bothersome and niggling in the back of my mind. The doctor checked me out and said, "Everything seems fine, but let's go ahead and do a lab test, just to make sure nothing's there." Okay, no sweat. Then, three days later, I get a message on my phone: "This is Amy from Dr. Melco's office. Could you please call me about your test results?" My heart skips a beat, and then the dialogue in my head goes something like this: "Oh, it's probably nothing. I'm sure they call everyone. She sounded so serious, though. If it was nothing, wouldn't she have just said so on the message? Geez, I can't get sick now, I've got too much to do. As if you can schedule getting sick—get over yourself. John [my husband] doesn't need this right now—he's got enough on his mind. I'm not going to even mention it. You know what—it's Friday. What is she going to say that's important today anyway? If it's bad, I'll just worry and it will ruin the weekend and if it's good, it doesn't matter anyway. I'll just call back Monday."

But then another manic Monday appears, and I forget to call. Tuesday's even worse, and I finally remember to call, but darn it, it's after five o'clock and too late. Wednesday I have meetings all morning and when I get finished there's another message on my phone, "Taylor, this is Amy. Please call Dr. Melco's office about your test results." Here we go again . . .

"She called back so it must be bad. She wouldn't bother if it were nothing. Now you're just being silly—she's just being helpful. Of all people, you should know that's what a doctor is supposed to do. *Stop!* Stop being stupid and just call her!"

So I call. "Hi, Amy, you left me a message about my test results?"

"Hi, Taylor, just wanted to let you know that the test was negative—everything seems fine. Dr. Melco said that if you start seeing the symptoms again, come in right away so she can get you checked out. Have a great day."

I can find a thousand good reasons why I put off returning that call, but the truth is, I was afraid.

Every test, every exam, every nagging symptom sends a shiver of fear down our spines and helps our monsters grow a little bit bigger. The key is to keep any risks, whether real or hyped, from clouding your judgment about your health. It's not closing that door that keeps the monster away; it's opening the closet, turning on the light, and looking that monster in the eye that will show him for the tiny creature he is.

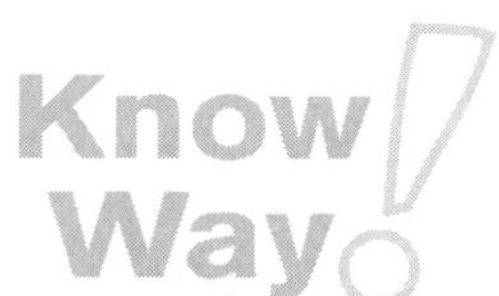

Rats and mice are the most dangerous animals on the planet. In the last thousand years, they have caused more deaths from disease than all wars combined.

Health fears are not like other fight-or-flight fears you might experience, but more often resemble feelings of dread or anxiety. They keep you up at night. They come out of nowhere when you're least expecting it. They leap out at you from the pages of the newspaper and your television screen. But you don't have to be held captive by the monster in the closet. By facing him and taking charge of your health you will quickly discover how easy it is to decrease your risks, be prepared for battle, and be armed with the right weapons to fight that monster if he ever does attack. The first step to taking charge of your health is to admit those fears, recognize how they affect your behaviors, and figure out how to open that closet door to bring that monster out into the light.

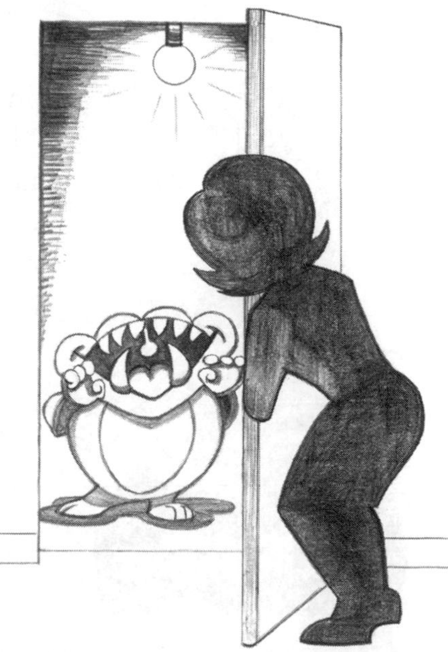

What's Your Health Character?

What do you become when it comes to your health? I call this your Health Character. Do you bury your head in the sand and ignore all the signs, or do you bully your doctor with your own diagnoses and cures? Do you hide under the covers at the least little scare, or do you have it all together? See if you recognize yourself in any of the following Health Characters.

Chicken Little

"I'm going home early today. I think I have a kidney infection."

I looked up from my computer at my colleague Monroe.

"A kidney infection?" I asked. "What makes you think that?"

"I've got an ache in my lower back, right where my kidneys are. And my wife gets kidney infections all the time and I've got the same symptoms."

Now, I knew that what Monroe's wife suffered from was occasional bladder infections, which are fairly common in women. I suggested that maybe Monroe's lower back ache was the result of him moving furniture over the weekend in his wife's redecorating project.

"Nope," Monroe winced, "it's definitely a kidney infection. I think I better head over to the emergency room."

"Okay," I sighed. "Call me later and let me know if everything's okay or if you need anything."

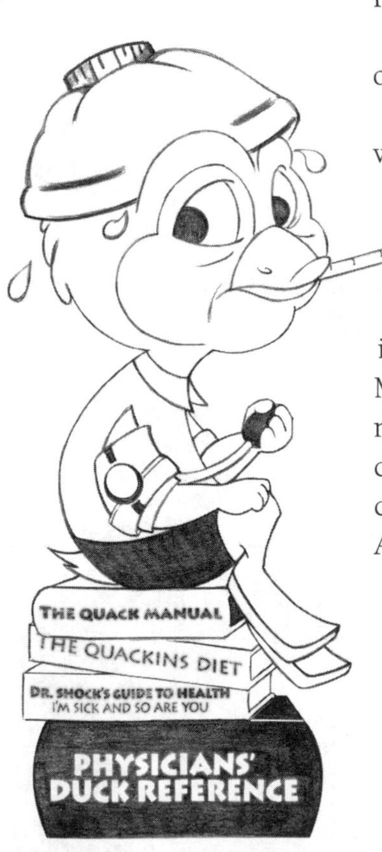

Now, I wasn't trying to minimize his symptoms or keep him at work, it's just that Monroe had earned enough emergency room frequent flier points to circle the globe a couple of times. If Monroe watched a TV show about heart disease, he was sure to show up the next day complaining of pain shooting down his left arm. Seeing a report on the Internet about cell phones causing brain tumors sends Monroe to his doctor demanding another MRI. And heaven forbid someone he knows get diagnosed with an illness. Monroe will be on the phone to his doctor quicker than a skunk can clear a room! Monroe couldn't seem to distinguish what was cause for real concern and what was just normal anxiety run amok. And like most Chicken Littles, Monroe also had a little duck in him, too (quack, quack). He would latch onto every crazy health story he could find, no matter how obscure or outlandish, searching for hidden symptoms and trying out the latest miracle cure. There was the book he bought that guaranteed a natural cure for every disease under the sun, including diabetes, heart disease, and cancer, by eating supernatural herbs and spices. Then there was the time he brought in grapes soaked in gin for everyone to try, promising they would ward off cancer. I don't know about the health benefits, but needless to say, our staff meeting that afternoon was pretty lively.

Everyone has a little Chicken Little inside imagining that the pain in your arm is from a heart attack or seeing a report on skin cancer and looking at every mole on your arm as a deadly lesion. But taking these fears too seriously can put a strain on both your spirit and the health care system. A phenomenon doctors call the Bill Clinton Effect showed how much Chicken Little is a part of our nation's health character. On September 3, 2004, former president Clinton made the news with reports of chest pains resulting ultimately in his having life-saving heart surgery. Doctors around the country saw a sudden surge in calls from patients with chest pains and heart attack worries. Emergency Medical Associates reported a 76 percent spike in ER patients complaining of chest pains on September 7 alone! While this kind of reaction can put a big strain on our health care system, the Chicken Little effect isn't all bad. President Clinton's openness in discussing his condition and treatment saved the lives of thousands who might never have been diagnosed.

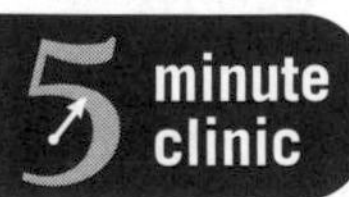

7 Things to Do When You Are Diagnosed

1. **Don't panic.** You will undoubtedly feel overwhelmed at first, but whatever the diagnosis, realize that medical technology has never been better. And know that the sooner you move on to treatment, the sooner you will feel better and be able to live your healthiest life.
2. **Don't let your doctor get you down.** It's your doctor's job to give you the facts and statistics about your condition, but remember they are just that—statistics. You're a real, live, breathing person with individual circumstances.
3. **Take time to feel your emotions.** It's okay to be mad, scared, frustrated, and any other emotion you feel. Give yourself time to feel those things and then move on to getting informed, taking action, and getting better.
4. **Get all the information.** Getting informed about your condition, your health, and the available treatments is what will save your life. Don't just depend on one doctor's opinion of how to treat your condition. Use the Internet, read medical journals, go to the experts in the field. Be proactive and take no prisoners. No one's going to do it for you.
5. **Don't make a snap decision.** Don't decide on a treatment plan until you get enough information. And make sure that you have a doctor who is experienced with your condition.
6. **Stay positive.** People who successfully manage health conditions credit a positive attitude with being vital to living well and feeling better.
7. **Live healthy.** Your body needs all its strength, so start eating better, be physically active when you can, and don't neglect the other parts of your healthy life.

By the same token, visiting your doctor on a weekly basis might help you catch some conditions early. But worrying about your health all the time and imagining that every symptom is a disease can make you (and even your doctor) ignore the bigger picture of your health. Looking for miracle cures can waste time, energy, and money on things you don't need that won't really do anything to make you feel better. Seeing your own demise in every celebrity death can lead you to worry about things that might never affect you and ignore actual health risks you might face.

Chicken Little Help Strategies

If you have some Chicken Little traits, try these strategies for refocusing your health energies in a positive way:

- **Understand your overall health picture.** Get a real picture of your health. Know your family risks, your own health history, and your healthstyle choices to understand what's worth focusing on and what may be an unfounded worry.
- **Ditch the mystery.** Fear of the unknown is what makes most of us cringe. Getting the right preventive tests and exams will take away the mystery and help calm your fears.
- **Steer clear of the "quack attacks."** Instead of wasting time and efforts on miracle cures or gimmicks, talk with your doctor about simple everyday things you can do to feel better and live longer.

And Monroe? He called me at home that night and told me that the emergency room doctor reported that his test results were negative and he had probably just strained his lower back. "But," Monroe continued, "while I was sitting in the ER waiting area I was talking to another patient there with a rash on his arm. I don't want to worry you, but I've been feeling itchy and I think it might be . . ."

RESOURCE

Reliable Health Information Online

Some great sources for unbiased health information are at www.berkeleywellness.com and www.mayoclinic.com.

Ostriches

The Ostrich is the Health Character that many people, especially if you're relatively healthy, can easily identify with. The ostrich is a character that buries its head in the sand and hopes for good luck to keep healthy. Self-treaters, ostriches often wait until their feathers are falling out to find out if something's really wrong.

Take Maria, for example. She's a classic Ostrich. Maria is thirty-eight years old, married, with three young boys. Maria's little purple monster is one many women would recognize—breast cancer. Like mine, Maria's mother was diagnosed with breast cancer in her forties, and although she was successfully treated, that history sets off a big red flag for breast cancer risk in the daughters of these women. That monster may wear a pink ribbon and go on a lot of walkathons, but it's still there lurking in your closet every day. Maria told me one day how she shuts that closet door and turns out the light . . .

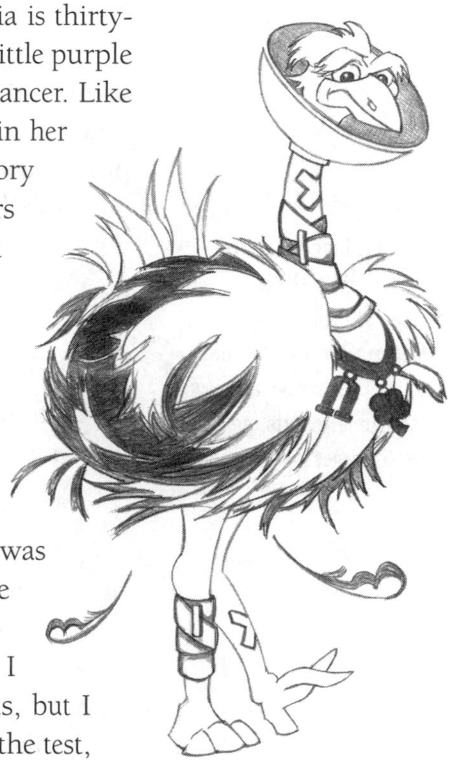

> I get too scared hearing all those statistics. I just dread the moment at the doctor when I'm giving my family history and they say, "Any cancer?" As soon as I say, "Yes, my mother had breast cancer when she was forty-two," their face just drops and they start telling me how I've got a one-in-four chance of getting breast cancer and how important mammograms and exams are. I feel like I'm sick already! I know it sounds ridiculous, but I have this superstition that if I go to the doctor or have the test, they'll just find something bad, so I just don't go. Anyway, who's got the time to get sick? I just can't think about that. To tell you the truth, I'd rather tune it all out. I figure I'm going to live the best I can and just deal with it when it happens.

This Ostrich behavior, while very common, is not just dangerous, but deadly. The worst part is that Maria's fear is keeping her from doing the very things that could save her life one day. A history of breast cancer in your family is not a death sentence, but ignoring that risk could very well be.

Now here's what the Ostrich overlooks. It's true that statistically the average woman has a one-in-eight chance—about 13 percent—of getting breast cancer during her lifetime. If you have a close relative who's had the condition, those chances go up to about one-in-four—around 25 percent. But that also means that the average woman has an 86 percent chance of *not* getting breast cancer. That's seven out of eight women who won't get breast cancer in their lifetimes. And even Maria, at 75 percent, is much more likely to hear good news than bad when she visits the doctor—*if* she visits the doctor. By ignoring her risk and avoiding preventive visits and screenings, she lowers her odds for early diagnosis, positive treatment, and even survival, if breast cancer ever does surface. On the other hand, even if Maria does get a breast cancer diagnosis and is proactive in her treatment, the odds are heavily in her favor that she'll go on to live a long, healthy life. That's where the Ostrich has it wrong. Avoiding your health instead of taking action doesn't make it go away and may, in fact, make your worst fears come true.

RESOURCE

Unbiased Health Reporting

Check out Consumer Reports' On Health newsletter. Subscribe at www.consumerreports.org/cro/health-fitness/index.htm.

Ostrich Help Strategies

If you find the Ostrich familiar, try these strategies to help you get more involved in your health before it's too late:

- **Get a Health Buddy.** Find someone (another Ostrich is great) to be your Health Buddy. Work together to develop plans for your health and then give each other encouragement to stick with your plan. Schedule checkups together, help each other take a health assessment, and offer support along the way.
- **Don't just hope for the best, find it.** Hoping for the best is just silly when it comes to your health. Finding out your risks won't make them any more risky, but it will let you know what you can do to minimize them and live your healthiest life.
- **Don't turn off the noise, just turn it down.** Don't ignore every health story you see or avoid the subject when it comes up. Being informed is never a bad thing; just try to keep it all in perspective.

The Bulldog

Weary after a day packed with patients, Dr. Natalia Meeks looked at her appointment schedule for tomorrow. Seeing a name she recognized at the top of the list, she shouted out front to Betty, her receptionist, "Is Mr. Reilly really my first appointment of the day tomorrow?"

"Yep," Betty shouted back. "You know he says that the first appointment is the best of the day because that way you won't keep him waiting and you'll be fresh."

"I'll be fresh all right," Dr. Meeks thought. It wasn't that she disliked Mr. Reilly; in fact, as far as patients went, he could be pretty interesting. It was just that his appointments took up a lot of time, and often she felt like she'd been a little bullied after he left, without really doing much for his health. "Better not schedule anyone else for that early-morning slot, Betty."

"Already done, Dr. Meeks."

Mr. Reilly is a Bulldog. Determined not to be at a disadvantage, he charges into the doctor's office armed with Internet stories, pages from medical journals, and his own diagnosis and treatment plan before Dr. Meeks can even put on her stethoscope. Instead of viewing his doctor as a partner in his health, he sees her merely as someone to sign his prescriptions, order up the tests he wants, and validate his diagnoses. Whenever Dr. Meeks sees one of those drug ads on television that ends with someone walking in a field while the narrator says, "Ask your doctor if this drug is right for you," she always smiles and thinks of Mr. Reilly, because he will definitely ask if the drug is right for him—even if he doesn't quite know what it is for.

The Bulldog's strategy is that a good offense is the best defense—being aggressive about your health is the only way to get good care. It's understandable where this philosophy comes from. Left on our own to manage our health, many of us have had to become our own health advocates. Doctors no longer have the time or the opportunity to be your family doctor, knowing your history and anticipating what you might need. Often you're on your own to determine which specialists to see and when, what procedures to have and which treatment option to choose. If there's one lesson to be learned about health in the twenty-first century, it's that you're in charge whether you like it or not.

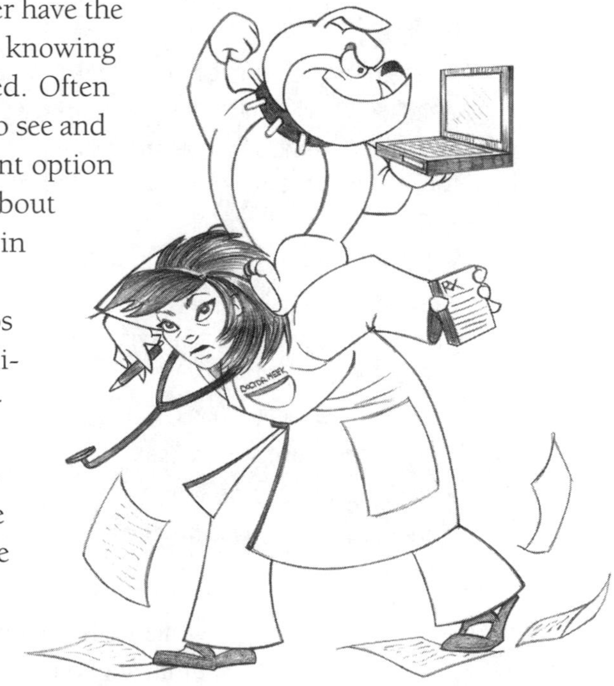

The easy availability of medical information helps bring out the bulldog in us all. Added to the old reliable sources of magazines, television, and newspapers comes the ability to search the archives of medical journals, universities, and scientific organizations online, helping many patients know more about their conditions, new drug therapies, and the latest research results than their doctors.

But the old proverb "A little knowledge can be a dangerous thing" is never more true than when it comes to your health. There's a fine line between taking charge of your health and biting off more than you can chew. A good doctor will be a partner in your health and can use her years of practical experience to help you put things in perspective, make a levelheaded evaluation of tests and treatments, and dig through the mountains of information and marketing to find what's right for you.

Internet 9-1-1

Fewer than half of the consumers who say they researched health conditions on the Internet came away with a better understanding of their health condition or how to treat it. Try some of these tips for better success on the Internet.

1. Make sure search terms are more restrictive.
   - Search for *hypertension + weight* instead of just *blood pressure* to find out how your weight affects your blood pressure.
   - Use Advanced Searching to restrict the date and get more current information.
2. Go directly to Web sites you know are reliable.
   - Universities (hopkinsmedicine.org)
   - Hospitals (mayoclinic.com)
   - Medical journals (jama.ama-assn.org)
   - Government entities (nih.gov, fda.gov, cdc.gov, healthfinder.gov)
3. Look at foreign sites for a new perspective on a health issue.
   - Canada (hc-sc.gc.ca)
   - Britain (patient.co.uk)
4. Understand that sites (especially commercial ones) may omit some information, such as:
   - certain treatment options
   - new or controversial treatments
   - homeopathic options
   - treatments contrary to their bias

Bulldog Help Strategies

If you find some Bulldog surfacing in your dealings with doctors and other health professionals, try these strategies to help smooth things out:

- **Find a doctor you respect.** Having a doctor you intimidate or don't trust won't do either of you any good. Find someone you respect to form a mutually beneficial relationship.
- **An ounce of skepticism is worth a pound of cure.** Don't believe everything you read on the Internet or see on television about health. Always ask yourself what they are selling you to understand where the information is coming from.
- **Patient, don't heal thyself.** You do need to manage your own health, but don't do it without getting professional advice. A good doctor will use experience and expertise to recognize when symptoms hint at something more serious and help you keep your health in check.

The Fox

The Fox is the health consumer we'd all like to be. Well informed and well prepared, the Fox understands her health conditions and how to manage them to live life to the fullest. Her relationship with her doctor is one of mutual trust and respect. She understands that while he is the coach, sketching out plays and giving direction, she is ultimately on the field as the quarterback, and it's up to her to carry the ball to the goal line. The Fox has a plan for her health that includes not only preventive screenings and regular checkups, but goals for her overall health, eating, exercise, and lifestyle choices. She approaches any health challenges she might face with an informed, positive outlook to find out as much as she can about the treatment options available in order to evaluate which treatments fit her priorities and her life.

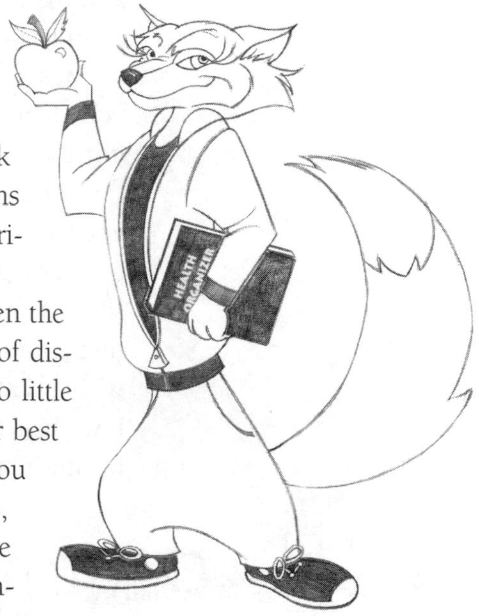

But even for Foxes, health isn't an idyllic paradise. Even the best Foxes among us must exist in a health care world of disjointed organizations providing too much marketing, too little prevention, and too many mixed messages. Despite your best efforts to be an informed, take-charge health consumer, you will run into the doctor who doesn't present all the options, the lab that screws up your test results, the miracle cure you've just gotta try. In 2005, Dick Pettingall, CEO of Minnesota's largest hospital group, called for health officials to start rethinking how our health care system is run. "On 9/11, 3,000 people died tragically, but 45,000 died needlessly in hospitals last year and where's the call to action? We have to stop repairing and start redesigning the system." The key is to not get discouraged, get on top of your health, and realize that you must take charge of your health. You are the best-qualified and most motivated candidate for the job.

A Brand-new You

You may have parts of all of these characters or some more than others. Your Health Character may change depending on the situation. I've seen moms who are the fiercest Bulldogs you'd ever run into when it comes to their kid's health, but bury their head in the sand about their own well-being, and Foxes who have a great diet and exercise plan, but haven't had a checkup in ten years. What's important is to examine how you feel about your health, face your fears, and figure out what you're willing to do to feel better and live longer.

I can't guarantee that you'll never get sick or that you'll live to be a hundred. I can't even tell you that you'll enjoy going to the doctor! But I can promise you that if you use the eight prescriptions in this book, you'll change not only the way you feel about your health, but also the way you feel about your life. You'll approach your health in a completely different way. You'll find a new source of peace and power.

Most importantly, you'll be ready for any health challenges you or your family members face. You'll understand how to decide what's important, be empowered to demand the care you deserve, and feel the confidence and strength to make the decisions to keep you and your loved ones healthy and protect your lives.

It's surprising to note that people with different health conditions share some common side effects—emotional, not physical, as you might think. For example, one out of five people who are hospitalized with a heart attack will experience depression in the months that follow their attack, even if their prognosis is excellent and they can resume normal activities. This depression actually puts them at higher risk for another heart attack. Many people with diabetes experience depression, anxiety, and even panic as they cope with the daily demands their condition requires. These emotional conditions are caused by many complex feelings—believing that a condition is somehow your fault, fearing the unknown, and feeling out of control of your destiny, among others. As you discovered in your Health Fears Appraisal, a lot of fears can be hiding unanswered in your mind: How will this condition affect my life? Will I ever have my old life back and be able to do all of the things I love? Will I be able to work and pay my bills? How will my family handle this? Why did this happen to me? And, of course, will I die?

While these subjects may make you uncomfortable and you might want to "just not think about it," keeping those fears locked away is exactly what that little monster loves to eat. Shutting those fears in the closet lets the monster keep getting bigger, feeding on your fears, getting more and more powerful, until he grows into something truly scary.

Acknowledging and facing your fears can free your mind and let you move forward to take

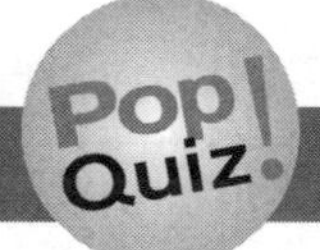

Strange Health Facts

1. Standing up too quickly after a meal can make your blood pressure drop. True False
2. Eating an orange with a steak is a good way to get more iron in your body. True False
3. Drinking water can prevent a heart attack. True False
4. One in four people sneeze when exposed to light. True False
5. Most heart attacks occur at night. True False

Answers

1. True. And it can cause dizziness and light-headedness, especially if you're age fifty or over.
2. True. Vitamin C helps your body absorb iron.
3. True. Men who drink at least five glasses of water a day have a 54 percent lower chance of dying from a heart attack than men who drink only two glasses. Tea, juice, coffee, and beer don't count!
4. True. Strange, but true.
5. False. Most occur between eight and nine in the morning.

your health back from that monster. Releasing your fears from the closet will release you and let you stop believing that you can't control your health, stop thinking that nothing you do will keep you from getting sick, and will empower you to take charge of your health and claim your health power, especially when you need it the most.

Even though medical news makes the headlines nearly every day, many of us ignore our health until something goes wrong, relying on doctors and the health industry to manage our health for us. In reality, millions of people unnecessarily get sick and die every year because they didn't take steps to do what they could to take charge of their health. From medical mistakes to drug reactions to undiagnosed conditions, we face a barrage of risks to our life and our well-being by not being proactive. How many of these seven mistakes are you falling prey to? Answer true or false to each statement in the box on pages 44–45.

Start Today

Before moving on to the next prescription, I want to talk about getting started on your health. Have you ever found yourself saying, "Tomorrow I'm going to . . . start eating better; start exercising; give up smoking; take better care of myself"? Well, I'm going to ask you to do something radical when it comes to your health. Stop talking about tomorrow. Do you know what happens in your mind when you say, "Tomorrow I'm going to . . ."? Tomorrow arrives and what does your mind think about? Tomorrow. Your mind isn't focused on what you're doing today.

I'm going to ask you to flip that statement around. When you find yourself saying, "Tomorrow I'm going to . . . ," I want you to stop and instead say, "Today I will . . ." Think for a moment about the power of that statement.

"Today I will."

Not sometime, but today. And not "I'm going to"—"I will." Now here's the great part. Since you're committing to doing it today, it's going to force you to do things that are reasonable—things that you can start doing today. Because too often taking better care of our health gets put off until tomorrow, then tomorrow, then tomorrow, until the tomorrow comes when we wake up and we've got a health condition or we're sick. Your body can't wait until tomorrow; it's

The 7 Biggest Health Mistakes: Are You Making Them?

1. **I am not prepared for emergencies.** **True False**

   Most people don't have time to think about their health and safety every day. By keeping your critical information updated and on hand, you'll have what you need in case of a natural disaster or medical emergency or for everyday medical care.

2. **I don't manage my medications.** **True False**

   It's estimated that 1.5 million people are injured every year by medication mistakes. Managing your medications is essential to protecting your health. First, make a list of all your medications, both prescription and over-the-counter. Second, always follow medication directions. Third, check every prescription or medication you are given to make sure it's correct. Last, if you have any side effects, get medical attention right away.

3. **I don't have a plan for my health.** **True False**

   Not knowing and not caring about your health isn't an option anymore. You've got to get the facts about your health and your condition, take action to get the care you need, make healthier choices, and make staying healthy a top priority in your life.

4. **I don't have a written family and health history.** **True False**

   Your health and family history is key to gauging your risk for nearly every health condition, from heart disease to diabetes to obesity. Doctors are too busy during office visits to ask, so it's up to you to bring it up. Do some research, keep a written record, and go over it with your doctor at your next visit.

5. **I don't communicate openly and honestly with my doctors.** **True False**

   "Most patients hide confusion from their doctors because they're too intimidated to ask for help," according to former U.S. Surgeon General Richard Carmona. Find doctors you trust and give them honest, complete information. Don't be afraid to ask questions, and make sure you understand the answers.

6. **I don't know where my health dollars go.** **True False**

   You're being asked to foot the bill for more and more of your care. Not understanding how much you really pay for care and not allocating your budget to the right places means your money isn't being well spent and you're not taking care of your health the way you

The 7 Biggest Health Mistakes : Are You Making Them?

should. Prevention doesn't just protect your body, it protects your bank account as well, warding off financial ruin from unexpected emergencies and illnesses.

7. **I will worry about my health tomorrow.** **True** **False**

   Don't play the waiting game. Don't wait to get a preventive test. Don't wait for a condition to get worse before seeing your doctor. And most importantly, don't wait for someone else to take care of your health. There is no one else who cares the way you do. Take the power, take the reins, and take charge.

trying to function today. "Tomorrow I'm going to" is what stalls you, waiting for perfection. "Today I will" is what moves you on to progress. That doesn't mean you don't have long-term goals, but you don't have to solve every problem, you don't have to make monumental changes, you just have to start . . . today.

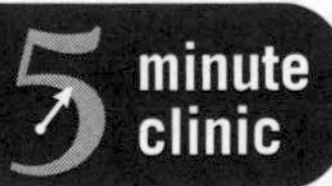

10 Things You Can Do Today to Be Healthier

1. **Drink more water.** Water nourishes every part of your body. And think how many calories you'll save by drinking water instead of soda or sugary drinks.
2. **Find out what your blood pressure is.** Stop at the drugstore or use an in-home test. This is one of the easiest measures to take and is a big indicator of your overall health.
3. **Write down one important thing about your health.** Your vital information, your health history, your family history: pick one and get started.
4. **Make a new friend.** Being a loner is not good for your mental health. Say hello to someone new and make their day, too!
5. **Turn your TV off for the day.** Not only will you be encouraged to get off the couch, but you'll avoid sensational health stories and commercials for fattening foods.
6. **Make an appointment for your yearly checkup.** If you've already got one scheduled, give yourself a pat on the back.
7. **Take a walk around the block.** You'll get vitamin D from the sunshine, breathe in fresh air, and get your blood flowing.
8. **Eat in.** Pack your lunch or eat at home. You'll save money and cut back on calories.
9. **Add three fruits and veggies to your day.** You want to shoot for six to eight servings, but adding three today will get you halfway there.
10. **Give someone you love a hug.** Physical contact is what feeds the soul. Everyone should get (and give) at least one good hug a day!

Taylor's Third Law of Health

Respect your doctors.
Don't worship them.

Prescription 2

Find a Great Doctor

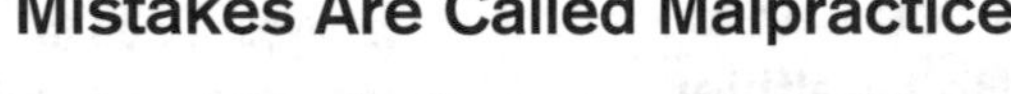

Mistakes Are Called Malpractice

In the movie thriller *Malice*, Alec Baldwin plays a brilliant surgeon, Dr. Jed Hill, being sued by a patient, portrayed by Nicole Kidman. In the film, Dr. Hill performed emergency surgery, removing both ovaries—without his patient's direct consent. While he did it to save her life, the operation leaves her unable to bear children. At a malpractice hearing Dr. Hill is asked if he has a "God complex" and he responds:

> The question is, "Do I have a God complex?" Which makes me wonder if this . . . lawyer, has any idea as to the kind of grades one must receive in college to be accepted to a top medical school? Or if you have the vaguest clue about how talented someone must be to lead a surgical team?
>
> I have an M.D. from Harvard. I am board-certified in cardiothoracic medicine and trauma surgery. I have been awarded citations from seven different medical boards in New England and I am never, ever sick at sea.

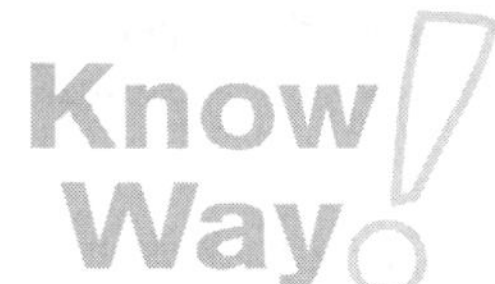

William McIlroy was the ultimate hypochondriac, undergoing four hundred operations at one hundred different hospitals. In 1979, he announced he was sick of hospitals and retired to a rest home, where he died four years later.

> So I ask you: When someone goes into that chapel and they fall on their knees and they pray to God that their wife doesn't miscarry or that their daughter doesn't bleed to death or that their mother doesn't suffer acute neural trauma from postoperative shock, who do you think they're praying to? Now you go ahead and read your Bible—and you go to your church and with any luck you might even win the annual raffle. But if you're looking for God, he was in operating room number two on November seventeen and he doesn't like being second-guessed.
>
> You want to know if I have a God complex? Let me tell you something—I AM GOD and this sideshow is over.

While Dr. Hill's answer is certainly dramatic and may not be indicative of most doctors, it illustrates a valid point. When your life or the life of someone you love is at stake, you want—no, *expect*—your doctor to be infallible. And every surgeon knows that when that scalpel is in their hand, in many ways, they do hold the power of life and death.

Critics of doctors like to cite this God complex—a characterization of physicians who act as if they are God, believing that they are always right, never make mistakes, and know everything. What you don't often hear is that being a god starts with someone worshipping you. If our doctors think they're infallible, it's in part because we expect them to be. In medicine, as in few other professions, mistakes are called malpractice and errors mean someone could die.

In truth, medicine, while called a science, is much more of an art. Some of the best diagnoses are made on a hunch—your doctor just looks at you or your test results and "knows" that something's not right. In medicine, as with much of life, there aren't always absolutes. What works for one patient may kill another. What one patient wants to hear may frighten or offend someone else. Putting someone on a pedestal makes them easy to look up to, but a little difficult to talk to.

> Physician—One upon whom we set our dogs when well and our hopes when ill.
>
> —AMBROSE BIERCE, AMERICAN SATIRIST

Between a Doc and a Hard Place

How well you get along with your doctor is more important to staying healthy than you might think. Dr. M. A. Stewart at the University of Western Ontario in London reports that when he looked at twenty-one independent studies, he discovered that how well you and your doctor communicate has a direct impact on your health—affecting your emotional health, the severity of your symptoms, indicators like blood pressure and blood sugar levels, and even pain.

And yet, for many of us, our relationship with doctors has never been worse. Surveys of consumers show we trust our doctors less and less, many times feeling as if they're more concerned with keeping costs down or making money than giving us the best treatment. And with pressure from health insurance companies to control costs, pharmaceutical companies to prescribe drugs, and their own families to earn a decent living, doctors are just as frustrated as we are. Fearing that any error will result in a costly malpractice suit, doctors are reluctant to admit they don't have an answer or made a mistake. One young doctor, I'll call him Cornell, told me how terrible he felt about a mistake he made:

> At two in the morning, a young mother came into the emergency room with her four-year-old son. Common middle-of-the-night, sick-kid symptoms: fever, vomiting, drowsiness. It looked like the flu to me and somehow, I just forgot to ask the child if his neck hurt. The mom showed me a slight rash that had developed, but again, I just missed the signals. Since the child was taking in fluids and the vomiting had subsided a bit, we gave him something to bring the fever down and sent them home. The next day I got a phone call I will never forget. I guess

How Well Do You Know Your Doctor?

Has your doctor ever . . .

- had malpractice insurance coverage denied?
- had hospital or surgical facility privileges revoked?
- faced disciplinary action by a hospital or credentialing agency?
- been refused participation as a provider in a health insurance plan?
- been convicted of a felony?
- been arrested for being under the influence of a controlled substance?
- had a malpractice lawsuit judgment against him?

How much do you know about the person in whose hands you place your safety, wellness, and even your life? Whether because we feel intimidated, are embarrassed to ask, or just don't think about it, we don't often know as much as we should about our doctors. Ask your health insurance plan, check with state accreditation agencies, and even ask your doctor, but get informed. Ask yourself, Would I ask these questions of a builder I was hiring to remodel my house or of an employee I was considering hiring? Then why not your doctor or surgeon?

the boy hadn't gotten much better overnight and the mom just "had a bad feeling," so she took him to his pediatrician in the morning.

"Damn it," the doctor ranted at me. "Where'd you get your training? Any med student could have diagnosed possible meningitis. Now the kid's going to have to come back in for an emergency spinal and you just better hope this doesn't get serious."

I was just getting off my shift, but I stayed on until the mom and boy got there. I didn't go in to apologize because I felt too bad, but I wanted to stay around and talk to the attending to make sure the boy was okay.

Well, it *was* bacterial meningitis, and the boy had to be admitted for treatment. He's fine . . . he came out of it okay, but that night still bothers me. I stopped in to see him one night when he was asleep and I just about lost it. I kept thinking what it would have done to that family if something had happened to that kid because of me. It was just stupid, lazy, whatever you want to call it—it was my fault for not asking the right questions. The mother kept asking me if I was sure it was just the flu, and I kept reassuring her. I have a daughter now who's three and I can't even imagine how mad I would be if that happened to her. The thing I feel the worst about is that I never did apologize in person. I asked one of the other doctors and they told me that it would just add insult to injury and give the family fuel for a lawsuit. No harm, no foul, they said. But I don't know, if it was me I would have liked to at least hear it from the doctor himself, that he was sorry. I was pretty cocky in med school, but I'll tell you what—even though I'd handled harder cases and probably made other mistakes along the way, that night really stuck with me.

What's in Your Doctor's Pockets?

Ever wonder what doctors carry around in those white coats? A recent poll asked doctors to empty their pockets to see what they were carrying. Here are the top items:

- Medical equipment, including stethoscopes, needles, pen lights, and calipers
- Pocket manuals of drugs and treatments
- To-do lists
- Telephone numbers
- Photocopied articles
- Prescription pads
- Personal digital assistants (PDAs)
- Calendars
- Handouts from lectures
- Treatment notes
- Family photos

And Cornell's not alone. Residents and doctors often suffer depression, guilt, and burnout as a result of making major medical errors, as reported in a study conducted on residents at the Mayo Clinic. One of the toughest parts is that there is no formal system in place for reporting, talking about, and fixing mistakes. Nearly half of the residents studied reported making major medical errors. While of course these errors often have major impact on the patients and their families, don't discount the negative impact it has on the doctors as well.

"Who cares?" you may ask. Well, even if we selfishly say we don't care about their feelings, it doesn't affect just them. It seems that the guilt and self-doubt lead to burnout, decreased compassion for patients, and even increases the likelihood that they'll make more errors in the future. The fact is, there is no system in place for allowing doctors to recognize their mistakes, and let's face it, in any system that depends on someone's judgment, mistakes can't be totally avoided. Since doctors can't admit the mistakes, nothing is done to make sure they don't happen again, and even more distressing, often a patient is left thinking that something went wrong for "no reason" instead of understanding that a mistake was made and getting action to correct it. This puts patients and doctors at odds: we mistrust them, and they regard every patient as a potential lawsuit.

Adding to this fractured relationship, every frustration we feel with our health system gets taken out on our doctors. The docs are on the front battle lines of health care, but don't feel they have much power,

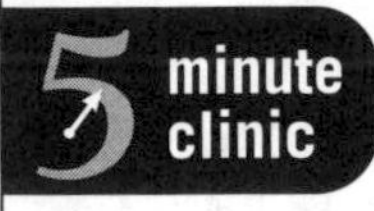

6 Things to Do if You Think a Doctor Made a Mistake

1. **Ask immediately.** Don't hesitate if you think something is wrong. A medical mistake can often be made worse by time or other procedures based on the wrong medication or treatment.
2. **Don't accuse.** Don't start taking names. Remember that your first priority is to find out if there has been a mistake and get it corrected as quickly as possible. You need everyone on the medical team to be on your side.
3. **Be forceful.** Remember that most doctors and hospitals don't have procedures for reporting and responding to mistakes, so they will often try to avoid rather than solve your problem. It's especially important to stand your ground if the patient is your child or someone else who cannot speak up for themselves. They need you to be their advocate and protect their life.
4. **Get a second opinion.** Ask a nurse, another doctor, or someone else to verify the treatment, medication, or diagnosis. Most medical errors are the result of one person's mistaken judgment or action, and by simply asking someone else to verify, you may catch the error before it has caused harm.
5. **Don't be embarrassed.** Don't worry about hurting your doctor's feelings or looking foolish. Medical mistakes happen by the thousands every day, so if someone tries to make you feel stupid, remind him gently of that fact.
6. **Don't threaten legal action.** Nothing will make doctors and nurses clam up faster than the threat of a lawsuit. Instead, focus on getting the situation corrected as quickly as possible. And honestly, until we all stop being so quick to point fingers when a mistake is made, we're not going to be able to stop them from happening at all.

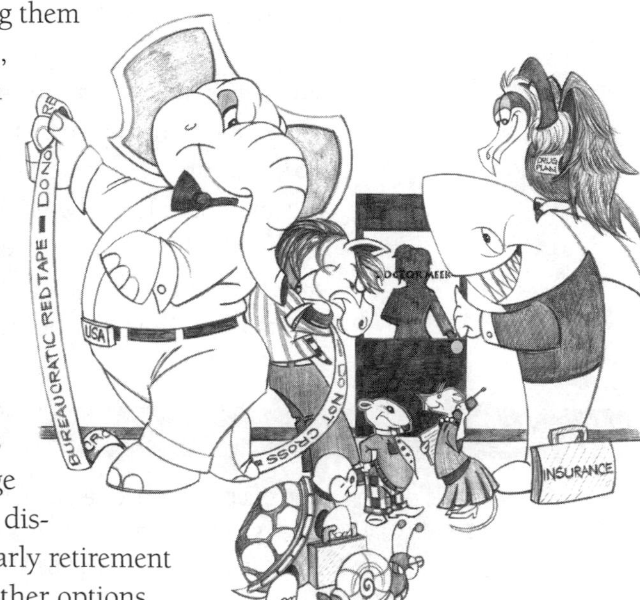

individually, to make things better, leaving them feeling frustrated. More and more often, their attention has been shifted away from care and toward the business of medicine and bureaucratic procedures. Every day they are besieged by insurance companies, drug company reps, and Medicare regulators, examining how they run their practice and coming between them and their patients. In one survey of physicians, 87 percent said their morale has gotten worse in the last five years. This creates a real threat to our health as large numbers of practicing physicians become disillusioned with their profession, taking early retirement or just leaving their practices to pursue other options.

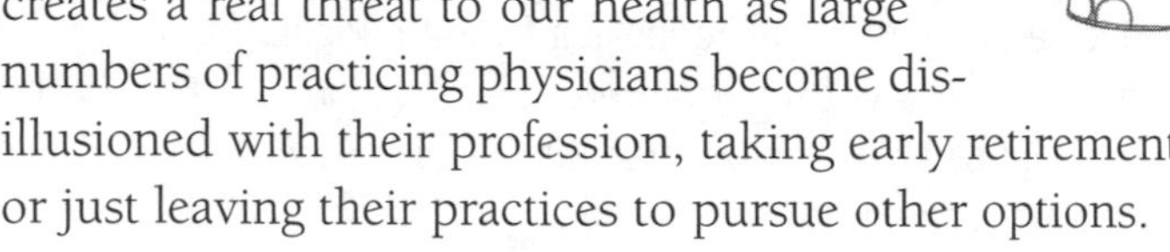

From Parents to Partners

Many doctors are also trying to figure out how to serve their patients as medicine has shifted from "doctor knows best" to care that is more focused on patients and what we need. Everyone agrees that involving patients more in their care is not only necessary, but also positive, but this shift has been tough for a lot of doctors to swallow. Involving patients in decisions about their health is not quite as easy as it sounds. Old habits die hard, and doctors often aren't taught the skills they need to build collaborative relationships with you. They might also think that they do involve you in the decisions, without being aware that they use technical terms you don't understand, make you feel rushed, or don't seem to want to hear what you have to say.

Are You Ready to Decide?

Determining how involved in decision-making you should be and want to be is harder for your doctors than you might imagine. It's hard to know for each patient how much they understand their situation and how much responsibility for making decisions they want to take. I myself got a wake-up call on that issue at a pretty young age.

My mother had suffered with back problems as long as I could remember. As is typical with back pain, most of the doctors she saw were stumped and just kept doing test after test and treatment after treatment that never seemed to work. She tried everything—acupuncture, chiropractors, traction, bed rest, exercise—and nothing did any good. Just when she had about given up, my brother, who was in medical school, suggested she see an orthopedic doctor he had worked with. Since the doctor's office was located about two hours away from our home and my mom's back often kept her from

Searching for Dr. Right

Fill out this short questionnaire to see what traits you're looking for in Dr. Right. Circle which trait you prefer in your doctors in each row. Remember that these choices aren't carved in stone. You might be able to find doctors who fit both sides, but it's more likely that you'll have to make some trade-offs.

I prefer a doctor with many years of experience who relies on traditional, proven treatments.	I would like a doctor who has more recent training and has been exposed to newer treatments and technologies.
I feel more comfortable with a doctor who takes charge of my care and tells me what to do.	I want a doctor who gives me the information I need, then lets me be in charge of my health.
I want a doctor who is sensitive and will consider my feelings when discussing my health.	I am looking for a doctor who is straightforward and does not beat around the bush.
If I were to get bad news, I want a doctor who would give me the truth over giving me false hope.	If I were to get bad news, I want a doctor who would give me hope over giving me the whole truth.
I want a doctor who prefers trying noninvasive treatments, like physical therapy, before recommending surgery.	I want a doctor who takes aggressive action, recommending the most advanced, cutting-edge technology available.
I prefer a doctor who is all business.	I want a doctor who is my friend.
I will use only a doctor who is board-certified.	It doesn't matter if my doctor is board-certified.
I want a doctor who meets my geographical, cultural, and gender specifications.	I want a doctor who is at the top of his field no matter where he is located, where he is from, or his or her gender.
I want a doctor who has all the answers and tells me what to do.	I want a doctor who is a good listener and is willing to educate me.

driving, I became her chauffeur and came to know Dr. Morgan so well that he eventually treated my own back problem, scoliosis. Dr. Morgan was great, the kind of doctor you dream about. First, he didn't dismiss my mother's problem as "all in her head," which many other doctors had. Second, he got right down to it. She had several ruptured disks and needed surgery to repair or remove them. My mom and I both breathed a sigh of relief. Finally, someone who was going to do something to fix her problem. Now, Dr. Morgan also wasn't one to mince words. "Back surgery is tough," he told us at one appointment. "You're going to need to do a lot of rehabilitation, have to stay in bed, and get a lot of help from your family until your back can heal. And remember, I can't guarantee it will work." Then he offered us an alternative treatment. "There's a new treatment that some doctors are trying where they inject a substance into the ruptured disk to try and dissolve the material that is irritating your spinal cord, causing much of your pain. We could try this treatment first, before we go in to remove any disks." Well, we did our part and researched the treatment. While it was new and fairly radical, it seemed that it had worked for a number of patients and had a shorter and easier recuperation, and my mother felt it was worth a try. The surgery would be a long one, so we had decided that I would drive my mother to the hospital the night before to check in and my father would come down in the morning and be there when she came out of surgery.

We got all settled in and I sat reading magazines by my mom's bedside as they came in to do the pre-op tests. Around eight that night, Dr. Morgan came into the room looking distressed. He proceeded to

Pop! Quiz! **Famous Docs**

1. Hippocrates, the father of medicine, pioneered the idea of patient confidentiality in 460 B.C. True False
2. A "Freudian slip" means you say something accidentally that you really mean. True False
3. Charles Drew, an African American doctor who pioneered blood transfusions, died when he was denied care at a white hospital after a car accident. True False
4. Jonas Salk, developer of the polio vaccine, worked his final years on a cure for AIDS. True False
5. The man who received the first heart transplant by Dr. Christian Barnard lived eighteen years after the transplant. True False

Answers

1. True. The Hippocratic Oath is still recited by doctors today.
2. True. Sigmund Freud was the father of psychotherapy.
3. False. This is a popular urban legend. Another doctor who was in the accident with Dr. Drew says they were all given excellent care.
4. True. Jonas Salk died in 1995 at the age of eighty.
5. False. The patient lived only eighteen days, succumbing to pneumonia caused by the anti-rejection drugs he was taking.

tell us that one of the tests had indicated that there was a risk that my mother might have an allergic reaction to the substance that was to be injected into the disk (a small percentage of patients did) and that the result could be serious, even death. There seemed to be no way to test conclusively for the allergy beforehand, but a preliminary test had put her in a range with a slight risk. After giving us the information he said, "I'll let you two talk about it and I'll come back in about an hour and see if you want to go forward with the surgery."

I looked around the room—"You two" who? Me? At seventeen I was expected to help my mom make this life-and-death decision? We called my dad and brother, but of course, since they weren't there it was difficult to ask them to make a long-distance decision. Even though my brother was a medical student, this wasn't his area of expertise, so he was working off only a little more knowledge than we had. Basically it came down to a decision-making process that people deal with in hospitals every day: weigh the benefits against the risks. I just kept thinking that someone in this hospital must be more qualified than I was to help my mother make this decision. I even went out into the hall, found Dr. Morgan, and asked him for help.

"I can't tell your mom what to do," he said. "Besides, I've seen how you've helped your mom before. She trusts you. There's no one in this hospital who cares about your mom the way you do. There are risks to both surgeries. I can give you the facts, but you have to help your mom make the decision that's right for her."

I went back into the room. My mother asked, "What do you think?"

"Well," I said, with all the authority I could muster, "this is a pretty new treatment and it's not like there are no other options. I just can't see taking this risk with your life. I say we pass and go home and go ahead with the regular back surgery on your disks."

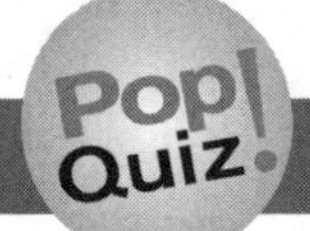

The Flu

1. Peak flu months are June through October. True False
2. The flu virus undergoes a major change every ten years. True False
3. Antibiotics are the most effective treatment for the flu. True False
4. You should not get a flu shot if you are allergic to eggs. True False
5. The flu mostly affects your circulatory system. True False

Answers

1. False. Peak flu months are December through March.
2. True. Since most people don't have immunity to the new strain, this mutation can cause epidemic outbreaks.
3. False. Antibiotics don't work against the flu. The best treatment is to treat your symptoms and get plenty of fluids and rest.
4. True. The flu vaccine is grown in chicken eggs.
5. False. The flu primarily affects your respiratory system.

My mom said, "I think so, too. I'd rather have the easier surgery, but I think the risk is a little more than I'm willing to take."

Dr. Morgan came in the room and we told him our decision. "I'm so glad," he said. "You didn't show a very big risk, but it's enough to give me pause. I couldn't in good faith tell you not to do it, but I just feel better taking the safer road."

I glanced up from packing up my mom's things as Dr. Morgan left the room. He gave me a little smile and nod as if to say, "Good job."

While that was a tough decision for us, it was a tough call for Dr. Morgan, too. Were we ready to make the decision ourselves? Should he trust his instincts and keep us from this new technique, or was he just worrying too much because he was a caring doctor? We often like to think that medicine is an exact science where the answers can all be found in a statistical chart, but unfortunately, that's not always the case. Judging how ready—and how qualified—a patient is to make a major decision, or even a small one for that matter, is not always obvious.

So it's obvious that your doctor shouldn't be performing procedures on you without getting your permission. "Informed consent" is a legal requirement recognized by all ethical doctors. But making sure you understand, help decide on, and embrace treatment decisions—called "valid consent"—is murkier.

This doesn't mean that the doctor can't put in her two cents. It's perfectly ethical and desirable for your doctor to express to you her opinion and the experience she's had with other patients. In fact, one of the most useful questions you can ask a doctor is, "What would you do if this were you (or your mother, or your child)?" If you've got a physician who tends to be detached from his patients, this can jolt him back to your space and get him to put himself in your shoes, considering how different treatments might actually affect his life. It's okay for doctors to try to persuade you, but not okay for them to

Getting Your Consent

What Doctors Should Do to Help You Decide

Valid consent means that you understand your options and have chosen the option yourself. Six general guidelines that responsible doctors follow are:

1. Information is presented in a way that you can easily understand.
2. You're given a full, clear explanation of the procedure and the reasons for doing it.
3. You're told the expected benefits.
4. You're told the possible risks, including long-term effects, potential complications, and how the procedure might affect your condition and your life.
5. You're given the alternatives to the procedure in a balanced way.
6. You understand what might happen if you choose not to go forward with the procedure or to do nothing.

manipulate you, lie, threaten, or abandon you if you don't do what they want.

So if your doctor tells you, "I really wish we could work on a plan for you to stop smoking," that's great. He's not only doing his job, he's showing you he cares about you. Now if he refuses to treat you because you can't (or won't) stop smoking, that's not ethical behavior.

Paging Dr. Wrong

Despite the tough circumstances doctors work in, it's also a fact that there are just some bad apples out there. Some doctors don't listen;

Okay or Over the Line?

How do you know if a doctor's behavior or his words are inappropriate? A good guideline is that if you feel uncomfortable with a situation, there's a good chance it's not okay. Express your feelings to the doctor or exit the situation before anything harmful happens.

Okay

Asking you to disrobe and get into a gown while he or she leaves the room.

Appropriate touching related to giving you a physical exam. The preference is to have a nurse in the room for any uncomfortable examinations (such as pelvic exams or breast exams).

Asking you about personal situations that may be affecting your health and well-being (such as physical and emotional abuse, risky sexual behaviors, or healthstyle choices) in a nonjudgmental way.

Telling you about certain conditions associated with your ethnicity that you may be at a higher risk for (such as diabetes, heart disease, or genetic conditions).

Asking that you provide proof of insurance or ability to pay or prepay for office visits and treatments.

Over the Line

Asking you to disrobe while he or she is in the room or not providing you with an appropriate gown or cover.

Inappropriate touching not related to your exam.

Not forwarding your records to another doctor (even if you owe your doctor back payments).

Asking for a date or initiating a personal relationship outside the office.

Not telling you about available treatments that are not covered by your insurance or may be expensive.

Asking you to become involved in a business or financial deal.

Not telling you the risks and benefits associated with a medicine or treatment.

Making demeaning, racial, ethnic, or sexist comments.

Refusing you treatment in an emergency situation.

some doctors cut corners; some doctors even practice bad medicine (for example, lying to patients or deceiving insurance companies). You don't have to turn over too many rocks to find a physician with bad skills, bad motives, or both. Fiona, a woman I met at one of my health seminars, told me a tale I almost didn't believe . . .

> I was a college freshman and had been having ongoing bouts of bronchitis. The campus doctor sent me for a chest X-ray, but wanted me to see a specialist to be sure nothing was seriously wrong. I didn't have a doctor in the area, so I took his recommendation. With X-rays in hand I went to the pulmonologist's office. My first clue should have been when he put the X-ray in the viewer and goes, "Oh my god, there's a spot on your lung!"
>
> "You're kidding," I say, and he replies, "Actually I am, that's just a smudge on the X-ray."
>
> "Huh?" I thought. "Is he for real?" Well, then he comes over and listens to my breathing with a stethoscope. Okay, that's pretty normal, but then get this . . . he goes, "Are you promiscuous?"
>
> "What are you talking about?" I ask.
>
> "Well," he tells me, "maybe you're out in the cold air wearing low-cut blouses and sleeping around and that's why you keep getting colds."
>
> That's it. I grabbed my purse—luckily he hadn't asked me to put on a gown—and I was outta there! On the way out the nurse says, "Oh, Miss, what about your payment?"
>
> "Just try and bill me," I said as I slammed out the door. I actually wrote a letter to the AMA because I was so mad. The sad part is that I never did go to another doctor for my bronchitis because of that. It eventually cleared up after I moved to another part of the country, but I'm still pretty leery when I go to a doctor I don't know.

How to Fire a Doctor

- Avoid specific criticisms.
- Don't complain to your new doctor about your old doctor.
- Explain to your new doctor what you're looking for.
- Realize that the choice of a doctor is ultimately up to you.

Could a doctor really exhibit such bad behavior? You bet, although I believe that Fiona's experience is the exception, not the norm. Most of the physicians I've met are passionate about what they do, truly care about patients, and worry as much as we do about the problems of the health care system. How do you make sure you get one of the good ones?

It Takes Two

Just like any good relationship, the doctor-patient relationship must be a two-way street. We can't expect the doctor to read our minds (although that would be a good trick to teach in medical school). Now, I'm not advocating bringing out the Bulldog—peppering the doctor with hundreds of questions, giving him your theory not only on your condition but on world economics, and demanding the latest, most expensive, best-advertised treatment "As Seen on TV." I'm talking about figuring out what your needs and expectations are and communicating those needs to your doctor in a positive way. Many patients say that their doctors often make health care decisions for them despite their wish to have a role in those decisions. This may be because your doctor doesn't understand what is important to you or because you've chosen the wrong doctor for you. Use this Patient-Doctor and the Doctor-Patient Communication Appraisals to see how well you and your doctor are communicating.

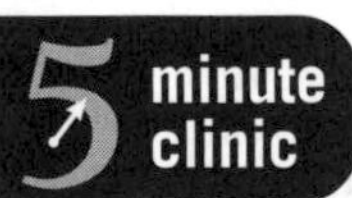

5 Principles to Being a Perfect Patient

Getting good care from your doctors is a two-way street. You should expect great service and care from your doctor, but you also need to take some steps to help them do their job to protect your life and keep you feeling good. Here are five principles that will help.

1. **Be prepared.** While doctors may want to spend an hour with each patient, in reality they can't do that and stay open for business. So come prepared with a written list of topics to discuss, medicines you take, and questions. Don't include the kitchen sink; limit it to your most important issues.
2. **Be pleasant.** Often when you see the doctor you don't feel well to begin with, but remember, they aren't to blame for your health issues (usually). So as much as you can, don't take out your frustrations with your health, your insurance company, your wife, your in-laws, or anyone else on your doctor.
3. **Participate.** Don't just sit there like a bump on a log. Ask questions, give information, and be an active participant in your health. Your doctor can't do it alone.
4. **Be proactive.** If your doctor gives you a treatment and you agree to it, stick with it. Doctors get frustrated when patients don't follow a treatment plan and then complain that they're not feeling better. If you don't like the treatment or can't follow it, tell the doctor before you leave the exam room.
5. **Treat them like a person.** Remember that doctors have families, worries, and aches and pains just like we do. Interacting with them person-to-person can improve your relationship and make you feel a little more human, too.

Patient–Doctor Communication Appraisal

How well do you communicate with your doctor?	Always	Sometimes	Never
1. Before I go to the doctor I prepare a written list of concerns and give it to my doctor.	3	2	1
2. I take a written list of the medications that I use, including over-the counter drugs, to my doctor visit.	3	2	1
3. I am honest about important issues with my doctor, such as smoking, drinking, and risky sexual behavior.	3	2	1
4. I ask questions about my condition and treatment until I understand everything.	3	2	1
5. I request written instructions about my condition and treatment plan or I take good notes.	3	2	1
6. I am honest with my doctor and myself about my willingness to make changes in my behavior.	3	2	1
7. I am able to communicate my symptoms to my doctor accurately and clearly.	3	2	1
8. I understand how the health care system works and how to use it when I need it.	3	2	1
9. I am calm and relaxed when discussing my health with my doctor.	3	2	1
10. I am willing to discuss my fears and feelings about my health with my doctor.	3	2	1

Scoring and Evaluation

Circling a lot of 3s means that you take pains to communicate what you need to your doctor. Check out the areas where you're circling 2s and especially 1s to see if the problem lies with your comfort level or with something your doctor is doing. You might also try taking a few steps to think about your health and prepare for your appointment before you go so that you are more at ease when you are there.

Doctor–Patient Communication Appraisal

How well does your doctor communicate with you?	Always	Sometimes	Never
1. My doctor talks to me on a level that I can understand and doesn't talk down to me.	3	2	1
2. My doctor is open and honest and doesn't keep information from me.	3	2	1
3. Before my doctor performs any test or procedure she explains exactly what is about to happen.	3	2	1
4. My doctor is always encouraging and never criticizes me.	3	2	1
5. My doctor acknowledges my concerns and objections and reacts accordingly.	3	2	1
6. My doctor makes me feel like I am a partner in my own health care.	3	2	1
7. My doctor knows my health and family history and uses it to improve my care.	3	2	1
8. My doctor takes the time to understand the problem that I am having with my health.	3	2	1
9. My doctor fully explains what he believes the condition is.	3	2	1
10. My doctor explains all of the available treatments and allows me to make an informed decision.	3	2	1

Scoring and Evaluation

Circling mostly 3s shows your doctor makes a real effort to communicate with you—she's a keeper! If you circled any 2s, you should talk with your doctor about how you might communicate better. A lot of 1s is a real cause for concern. If communication can't be improved, maybe it's time to look elsewhere for a doctor you feel more comfortable with.

How to Find a Doctor You Love

Finding the right doctor can be almost as important as finding the right mate. You're not going to get stuck picking up his dirty socks or holding her handbag while she's shopping, but let's face it, you and your doctors are going to be involved in some pretty intimate situations. You've got to trust each other, be totally honest about personal matters, feel comfortable about the boundaries of the relationship, and have the confidence to rely on them to help you make some of the most important decisions of your life. You've got to be compatible emotionally, physically, intellectually, and with your respective powers in the relationship. I'm reminded of an episode of the comedy show *Seinfeld* where the characters were discussing who has "hand" in a romantic relationship. Their agreement was that the first person to say "I love you" loses the upper hand in the relationship. Hapless George Costanza then embarks on a plot to try to get back his "hand" after blurting out his professions of love in a moment of weakness.

You don't have to plot to make sure you have the upper hand in the patient–doctor relationship, but in reality there is lots of "hand" shifting or power juggling that goes on in the relationship between you and your doctor. You (or your insurance) pay the doctor—your hand. The doctor has more medical training than you—his hand. You know more about yourself and your symptoms—your hand. The doctor has the white coat on and you've got on . . . that little paper gown—his hand. You get the point. The goal is to build a relationship where you work together as a team to both get what you need.

Top 4 Traits Patients Want in Doctors

1. Kindness
2. Competency
3. Willingness to involve patient in decisions
4. Time for care

Let's look at the five keys for building a successful relationship with your doctors:

1. Figure out what you need.
2. Know where to look.
3. Evaluate your doctors.
4. Communicate what you want.
5. Know what to expect when you're a patient.

1. Figure Out What You Need

One young woman, Kristin, told me about an experience that showed her how important it is to have the right doctor for you:

I was about four months into my pregnancy when I tripped and fell down a couple of stairs. It wasn't a big fall and I didn't hurt anything, except my dignity. I called my doctor and she said to come on in "just in case." But a strange thing happened at the doctor's office. While my doctor examined me she started to tear up. She told me that if we didn't try and stop the labor, I would probably lose the baby. When I asked if the fall had caused this, she quickly replied, "Oh no, I don't think so," which didn't make sense, but I wasn't exactly in the mood to ask a lot of questions. Lying in the exam room I was upset, but I also remember thinking it was odd that the doctor had started to cry. Frankly, it made me a little uncomfortable. I'm not a crier, especially in front of strangers, and to be honest, it made me feel guilty—like I wasn't being emotional enough. I was trying to make a lot of decisions while lying in a hospital bed hooked up to about ten monitors and was trying to get through the experience the best I could.

The doctor, who had a three-month-old baby herself, promised she would be back in about two hours and we would discuss the decisions I had made. During that time I was visited by her partner, who was much more matter-of-fact. He told me the chance of stopping the baby from coming was slim. I asked what he would do if I was his wife, and he said, "Honestly, if it were my wife, I would allow the delivery to proceed naturally and try again. Sometimes nature makes the choice for you. Taking extraordinary measures might put your health or your ability to bear more children in jeopardy without changing the eventual outcome."

Know Way!

A normal person can shrink by as much as one inch throughout the day because of compression of the spine.

When my doctor returned two hours later as promised, she told me that in fact nature had made the decision for me—the measures they had taken were not working and she didn't think further tries would be successful. She started to cry again.

It wasn't an easy experience, but I got through it okay and a year later I gave birth to a beautiful, healthy baby girl. When I went for a follow-up appointment after the miscarriage, I asked again if the fall might have caused it.

The doctor looked at me sheepishly and said, "Probably."

> I asked her why she hadn't told me before and she said, "I didn't want you to feel it was your fault."
>
> I realized that although I really liked her and the level of care she gave was outstanding, we just weren't compatible. First, I didn't want to be shielded from the truth. While her intentions were nothing but pure, it actually had given me a lot of sleepless nights trying to figure out what had gone wrong or if I was going to have problems with future pregnancies. Knowing that it was the fall would have dispensed with these questions right away. I never blamed myself. It was clumsy to fall, but I hadn't been doing anything dangerous—it was just an accident. And another thing, I appreciate that she was sad about what happened—I was sad, too, and believe me, I did plenty of my own crying. But I have to admit, it kind of freaked me out that my doctor was crying when she was delivering news to me—I need someone who is able to be a little less emotional. It's weird because I picked a female doctor in the first place because I wanted someone who would be more sensitive, but then it bothered me when she was too sensitive. It really made me see that you can't just have a "good" doctor, having the doctor who matches your needs is important, too.

The Doctor Wish List, beginning on page 64, will help you figure out what you need. Rank each factor on a scale from 1 to 3. It's highly unlikely that you will find the perfect doctor who will fulfill every wish on your list. Just like in other relationships, you've got to be willing to compromise or find trade-offs.

2. Know Where to Look

So where do you find a doctor you'll love? You sure can't pick her up at the local nightspot, and unfortunately, there's no match.com for doctors. That aside, there's lots of easy ways to start getting the skinny on some doctors who fit the bill.

Health insurance directories A listing in a health plan directory isn't necessarily a recommendation from the plan, but it can be a good place to start looking. Many plans do things like check credentialing and board certification, check for malpractice suits and other

Your Doctor Wish List

	Doesn't Matter	Kind of Matters	Major Biggie
Skills			
1. A doctor who can treat everyone in my immediate family.	1	2	3
2. A doctor with a particular specialty.	1	2	3
Specialty ____________________ (see Reference Guide for list)			
Credentials			
1. Educated at Ivy League or prestigious medical school	1	2	3
2. Completed residency or worked at major medical center (such as the Mayo Clinic or Johns Hopkins)	1	2	3
3. Board-certified in specialty	1	2	3
Experience			
1. Been in practice ten years or more	1	2	3
2. Been in practice five years or more	1	2	3
3. Recent graduate experienced with latest treatments	1	2	3
4. Experienced in particular procedure	1	2	3
Procedure ____________________			
Learning			
1. Keeps up-to-date on latest treatments, technologies, and drugs	1	2	3
2. Seeks out clinical trials for patients to participate in	1	2	3
3. Relies on tried-and-true treatments	1	2	3
4. Open to use of alternative or homeopathic treatments	1	2	3

May be more important when choosing a specialist than for your general care physician. (→ Credentials item 2)

If you're having a procedure, find out how many times the doctor has performed it. (→ Experience item 4)

If you've got a condition like cancer and want to get into a clinical trial, make sure the doctor is tuned in to those. (→ Learning item 2)

Your Doctor Wish List

	Doesn't Matter	Kind of Matters	Major Biggie
Affiliations			
1. Has privileges at particular hospitals	1	2	3
Hospitals ________________			
2. Part of a group practice with other doctors in same specialty	1	2	3
3. Part of a large medical group with access to various specialists	1	2	3
4. Belongs to prominent medical associations (such as AMA and AAP)	1	2	3
5. Wide network of associates to make referrals from	1	2	3
Practical			
1. Specific sex of doctor (male or female)	1	2	3
2. Older doctor with more experience	1	2	3
3. Younger doctor with more recent education	1	2	3
4. Speaks specific language	1	2	3
Language ________________			
5. Certain office location (close to home or office)	1	2	3
Preferred location ____________			
6. Certain office hours (for example, weekends or evenings)	1	2	3
Hours needed ______________			
7. Can spend time with you during office visits	1	2	3
8. Can schedule same-day appointments	1	2	3
9. Can schedule "sick" appointments within one or two days	1	2	3
10. Can schedule "checkup" appointments within one or two weeks	1	2	3

(continued)

Don't be embarrassed if you prefer a male or female doctor. The key is for everyone to be comfortable.

Keep an open mind. Despite perceptions, studies show that older, more experienced doctors are not always the best qualified. And younger doctors may understand newer treatments, but might not have the experience in diagnosing conditions.

Highly sought-after physicians may be difficult to get an appointment with, but could be worth the wait.

Your Doctor Wish List (continued)

	Doesn't Matter	Kind of Matters	Major Biggie
11. Accepts certain insurance Insurance ____________________	1	2	3
12. Accepts patients without insurance	1	2	3
Relationship			
1. Traditional relationship—doctor leads and you follow	1	2	3
2. Partnership—you and doctor share in making decisions	1	2	3
3. Consultant—you lead in decisions and get information and support from the doctor	1	2	3
4. Doctor who is willing to let you set agenda for care	1	2	3
5. Doctor who has similar goals for your health	1	2	3
6. Courteous and helpful office staff	1	2	3
7. Nurses or physician's assistants available to answer questions	1	2	3
8. Doctor available to answer emergency calls	1	2	3
9. Answering service available to answer calls	1	2	3
10. Doctor willing to communicate via e-mail	1	2	3
11. Doctor comfortable with you seeking second opinions	1	2	3
Your Beliefs and Boundaries			
1. Doctor who shares your beliefs and values about:			
medical treatment	1	2	3
religion	1	2	3
end-of-life issues	1	2	3

Some doctors welcome second opinions and others get offended. Find out if the doctor is comfortable with it.

It's possible to have a positive relationship with someone who doesn't share your beliefs, but be open about them and be aware that clashes can surface.

Your Doctor Wish List

	Doesn't Matter	Kind of Matters	Major Biggie
patient involvement	1	2	3
alternative treatments	1	2	3
other ________________________	1	2	3
2. Doctor who supports your treatment boundaries including:			
blood transfusions	1	2	3
pain management	1	2	3
organ transplants	1	2	3
medication use	1	2	3
do-not-resuscitate orders	1	2	3
pregnancy termination	1	2	3
other ________________________	1	2	3

problems, and even do physical inspections to see if the doctor's office is presentable and if their office procedures meet minimum standards. If you don't have a health plan or can use doctors outside your plan, ask a colleague or a family member if you can borrow their directory to start looking.

Family members, friends, and colleagues Personal recommendations are probably the best way to find a doctor you'll like. You can get the scoop on what the doctor is really like and find out how they work. But remember that everyone has different needs from their doctors (we didn't fill out Your Doctor Wish List for nothin', ya know!), so listen carefully to what Aunt Millie says. She may describe a doctor who's perfect for you, but whom she just didn't like.

Doctors If you've got a friend or a family member who's a doctor, he can be a great resource for recommending good colleagues. They will give you the *real* story and can also ask around. Here again, you still have to rely on your own impression. Someone who's a great golf partner for your brother may just not suit your style when it comes to your asthma.

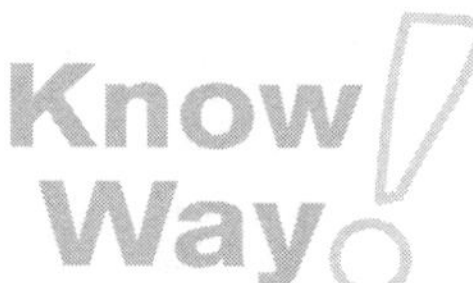

There are over 700,000 licensed physicians in the United States today. The number of family physicians fell more than 50 percent from 1997 to 2005.

Nurses Nurses are a great source of information about doctors and will usually be very candid about a doctor's qualifications, reputation, and personality. Nurses who work in hospitals can tell you who is good in their department and usually have a great network of friends and colleagues who can tell you the real deal.

RESOURCE

National Physician Directories

Directories for every medical specialty: www.nlm.nih.gov/medlineplus/directories.html

Online resources There are good resources for finding doctors online, but as with anything on the Internet, make sure you're using reputable sites and check what you find against other sources. The site in the sidebar to the right is a fantastic resource that lists the associations of virtually every specialty, with direct links to their sites to help you begin your search.

Newspapers, local directories, and phone books If you're shopping around for a new doctor, these local resources can be a great way to find doctors who are newer and may be looking to build their practices. You'll find both new and established doctors in the yellow pages, and doctors opening new practices often take out ads in the local directories (such as parenting guides or books for new home owners) and local newspapers. A newer practice may be just what you want if you're looking for more intimate, personalized service from a doctor who's trying to build his practice.

3. Evaluate Your Doctors

Whether you're looking for a new doctor or want to evaluate the doctor you have, use the compatibility test beginning on pages 69–70 to help you decide if you and your doctor are a match.

The First Date

Don't let your first appointment with a new physician be a blind date. Once you've written down the basic information you can get from a directory, a phone book, or an ad, give the office a call and get some additional information in a short phone interview. This will also give you a chance to interact with the office staff to see if they are courteous and willing to answer your questions or seem rushed and impatient. Remember, if they're not willing to answer your questions now, imagine what might happen when you need answers to a serious health concern!

Even if you've been seeing somebody for a while, it's good to take a step back and evaluate your relationship to make sure it is a positive

Are You and Your Doctor Compatible?

Basic Information

Physician name ______________________________

Specialty(s) ______________________________

Office location(s) ______________________________

Office hours ______________________________

Languages spoken ______________________________

Hospital affiliation ______________________________

Phone/fax/e-mail ______________________________

Is the doctor's specialty what you need?	Yes	No
Is the office location convenient for you?	Yes	No
Are the office hours convenient for you?	Yes	No
Is the doctor's hospital affiliation acceptable?	Yes	No

Phone Interview (conduct with office staff)

Office staff names ______________________________

Doctor's credentials and experience ______________________________

How long has the doctor been in practice? ______________________________

How long does it take to get an appointment for a checkup? ______________________________

How long does it take to get an appointment when sick? ______________________________

What is the fee for a routine office visit? ______________________________

Which insurance do you accept? ______________________________

Who covers when the doctor is not available? ______________________________

Is the doctor accepting new patients?	Yes	No
Does the doctor accept your insurance?	Yes	No
Is the doctor willing to schedule a "get acquainted" appointment?	Yes	No
Can I communicate with the doctor via e-mail?	Yes	No

First Impressions at the Doctor's Office

Office staff friendly and courteous?	Yes	No
Office staff organized and efficient?	Yes	No
Office staff happily answers any questions?	Yes	No
Office clean and pleasant?	Yes	No
Office crowded with waiting patients?	Yes	No

(continued)

Are You and Your Doctor Compatible? (continued)

Doctor Interview (ask doctor or complete based on your experience)

What are your goals for your patients? ______________________

What do you think of Internet health information? ______________________

How do you stay up to date on treatments? ______________________

How do you feel about second opinions? ______________________

Are your patients involved in clinical trials? ______________________

How can I reach you in an emergency? ______________________

What do you like most about being a doctor? ______________________

Your Other Questions

____

____

Doctor's answers ______________________

____

Did You Like the Doctor?

Did the doctor take the time to listen to you?	Yes	No
Did you feel comfortable asking the doctor questions?	Yes	No
Did the doctor answer in a way that you could understand?	Yes	No
Did the doctor ask you questions in order to get to know you?	Yes	No

If You Already Have a Relationship with the Doctor . . .

Does the doctor know your health and family history?	Yes	No
Does the doctor sit down and take the time to talk with you?	Yes	No
Does the doctor rush to prescribe a medication at every visit?	Yes	No
Does the doctor explain test results to you in a way you can understand?	Yes	No
Does the doctor give you treatment alternatives, explain each one, and give you a chance to evaluate them and make a decision?	Yes	No
Does the doctor give you educational material or tell you how to learn more about your health or condition?	Yes	No
Does your doctor tell you when you need follow-up care and what you should do if you continue to have symptoms?	Yes	No

Finally . . . Is It a Match Made in Heaven?

Do you like the doctor?	Yes	No
Is the doctor someone whom you trust and respect?	Yes	No

one for you both. Take a few moments at your next appointment to talk to your doctor about your relationship and your shared goals so you can evaluate whether it's a relationship you want to continue.

Divorce Court, Here We Come?

Even if you and your doctor fail the compatibility test, don't abandon the relationship right away. You may find that by mentioning some of your concerns to your doctor, you can nudge the relationship to be more open and productive for you both. If your doctor doesn't know, he can't correct the situation. It really isn't all that different from any relationship. Any marriage counselor will tell you that the most important thing is to recognize issues and find ways to improve communication. That's what this process is about—not criticizing your doctor or saying that you're a bad patient. It's about finding a patient-doctor match that will let you both be comfortable and enjoy the relationship and ensure that you get the right care and have the healthiest life possible.

4. Communicate What You Want

Okay, the work is done. You've found a doctor you respect, can communicate with, and trust to help you manage your health. Now you can just relax, sit back, and enjoy the ride, right? Not so fast. You make the majority of your health decisions in your everyday life—not sitting on that exam table in the doctor's office.

A recent study conducted in England shows that the average patient has as many as five agendas when they go to the doctor, with some patients having as many as twenty or more. While these agendas include things you would imagine, like symptoms, illness fears, diagnosis theories, and self-treatment questions, they also encompass issues such as emotional, social, and family problems. The sad fact revealed in the study was that only 11 percent of patients voiced all of their agendas when they saw their doctors. The most common agenda items left unsaid were worries about possible illnesses and what the future holds, patients' ideas about what is wrong, questions about medication and side effects, not wanting a prescription, and emotional issues. It was found that these unraised issues often led to problems, including medical mistakes, unwanted prescriptions, and patients not following treatments. Doctors in the study overestimated

What Patients Want to Talk About

Symptoms

Request for medication

Theory on diagnosis

Side effects

Health worries

Not wanting medication

How health is affecting their relationships

the extent to which their patients were concerned with medical treatment rather than with getting information and support. It seemed that unless the patients was obviously upset, doctors had trouble recognizing those who needed emotional support.

Doctors aren't oblivious to this fact. They are frustrated too when communication with a patient is poor. One of the doctors in the study commented, "I got so depressed when you described this man whose list of expectations went on to about eighteen points. . . . There's no way that I am ever going to be able to address even three of these, let alone eighteen." Another doctor labeled the man a "heartsink" patient—one who makes your heart sink because the communication just isn't working.

Communicating with doctors is a learned skill for most people, not something that comes naturally. Our medical system hasn't encouraged good patient-doctor relationships, so it's up to us to take charge and make it happen. Improving communication with your doctor is actually pretty easy. I'm going to give you some simple things you can do before, during, and after you get to the doctor's office to make sure you communicate exactly what you want.

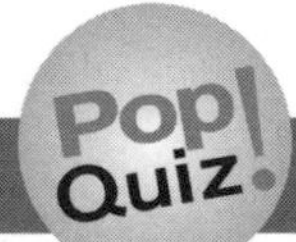

Know Your Phobia

1. Mageirocophobia is the fear of:
   a. magic b. cooking c. large groups
2. Suriphobia is the fear of:
   a. mice b. large groups c. celebrity babies
3. Ablutophobia is the fear of:
   a. Popeye b. bathing c. balloons
4. Anemophobia is the fear of:
   a. iron b. air c. cute fish
5. Dinophobia is the fear of:
   a. dizziness b. dinosaurs c. double vision
6. Gamophobia is the fear of:
   a. legs b. games c. marriage

Answers

1. b 2. a 3. b 4. b 5. a 6. c

Before You Go

Get prepared before you get to the doctor so that you can use your time and his time efficiently to get what you need. Prioritize what you want to accomplish at this visit—don't try to dump out the whole kitchen sink. Your doctor probably won't have time to deal with every issue, so decide what's most important for this visit.

Write down the details of your symptoms and be honest about what you've already tried to solve the problem, whether it's home remedies, your sister's prescription medication (not recommended!), or nothing at all. Take a little time to look up your symptoms at the library or on the Internet and develop a few ideas about what you think it might be. That doesn't make you a junior doctor, but it can help your doctor see which conditions you think most closely match your symptoms. Use the Going to the Doctor form on page 75 to help you prepare information about your symptoms so you can answer your doctor's questions and ask a few of your own.

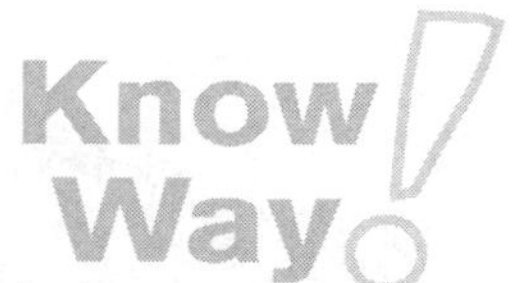

X-rays were discovered in 1895 by Wilhelm Röntgen. Virtually the same technology is still used today.

Have your health history organized and bring it to the appointment to help you answer your doctor's questions. The *Journal of the American Medical Association* estimates that information is missing in one out of seven office visits. This missing information is likely to adversely affect a patient 60 percent of the time, causing delays in care, mistakes, and unnecessary procedures or tests.

Bringing a Health Buddy or another person with you to your appointment can also help make sure you present all your information and get all your concerns answered. If you're not comfortable with someone else in the exam room, ask her to wait outside until the exam is completed and the doctor is ready to discuss what he's found. Even if having someone present during the discussion makes you uncomfortable, you'll know she is there in the waiting room in case you need support and someone to talk with after the appointment. Besides the moral support, she can help remind you to follow through with your treatments or any follow-up care you need.

Last, think about any questions you may have and write them down. The Going to the Doctor form gives you some suggestions. In truth, you'll probably come up with questions as you talk with the doctor, so you may want to carry a notebook so that you can jot anything down and make sure you ask about it before you leave. It's also a good place to keep notes about your doctor's diagnosis, treatment options, tests, or follow-ups you need to have.

6 Things You Should Do *before* Going to the Doctor

1. Decide what you want from the appointment. Prioritize your list.
2. Write down your symptoms and what you've already tried.
3. Get informed about your symptoms and what you think they could mean.
4. Bring your written health information. Include health history, family history, and medications.
5. Ask someone to go with you.
6. Write down questions for your doctor.

The Land of the "Ya-Buts"

You're prepared. You're informed. You're ready to step up and take control of your health. But there you are, sitting in the doctor's office, ready to be defeated by one tiny creature I call a "Ya-But." What's a Ya-But? You know, when your doctor says, "Georgia, you really need

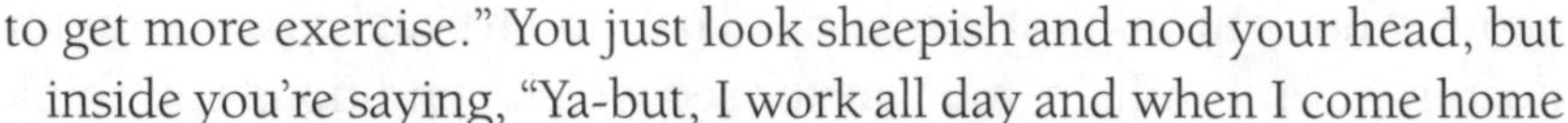

to get more exercise." You just look sheepish and nod your head, but inside you're saying, "Ya-but, I work all day and when I come home I have to help the kids with their homework, make dinner, and by then it's time to clean up the house and there's just no time." Or the doctor says, "Ed, I'm going to give you a prescription for a little something that will help you sleep." "Ya-but," you think, "I don't want to take sleeping pills; they make me groggy and I just don't want them." A Ya-But is that little guy who floats around in your head, keeping you from telling the doctor what you really want. I've said it before and I'll say it again: if the doctor tells you something you don't agree with or don't want to do—even if it's good for you—you must speak up and let her know. Nine times out of ten she will be glad you said something. That's the only way she can understand your priorities, your values, and the reality of your life to find a solution that you agree to, find reasonable, and can stick with.

There are five simple things you can do at the doctor's office to help you escape the Land of the Ya-Buts and get what you want.

1. **Be honest.** Tell your doctor what you want, what you're feeling, and what you're willing to do—and not do.
2. **Speak up!** Don't hesitate to ask your doctor the questions you've prepared, tell her about any hesitations or fears you have, or mention any other details she might find helpful in diagnosing and treating your condition.
3. **Be nice.** Kindness can go a long way in building a good relationship with your doctor and her staff.
4. **Be realistic.** Don't expect miracles. Don't even expect results if you're not willing to do your part. Remember that the choices are yours, but so are the consequences. If your doctor recommends simple changes that you choose not to follow, understand that your condition may worsen, meaning more radical treatments in the future.
5. **Be clear.** Make sure you understand what your doctor has told you before you leave the office. Review test results, make sure you understand treatment plans, double-check medication instructions, and know exactly what follow-up is needed. *If you don't know, ask!*

Going to the Doctor

Describe Your Symptoms

What are your general symptoms? ______________________

____

When did you first notice the symptoms? ______________________

How long have they lasted? ______________________

How severe are they? Mild Moderate Severe Debilitating

Do they come and go or are they constant? come and go constant

What treatments have you tried? ______________________

Did anything help? ______________________

What do you think is the problem? ______________________

Questions for Your Doctor

Doctor's diagnosis ______________________

What might be causing this condition? ______________________

Are these symptoms a sign of something serious? ______________________

Should I see a specialist? What kind? ______________________

How long will the condition last? ______________________

Is it likely to come back after treatment? ______________________

How can I prevent it from happening again? ______________________

What's the Treatment Plan?

Tests ______________________

Medications ______________________

Healthstyle changes ______________________

Physical therapy ______________________

Surgeries/Outpatient procedures ______________________

Other treatment ______________________

Appointment date

____

Time

____

Doctor

____

Reason for visit

____

____

____

____

Follow-up

Follow-up needed if:

____

____

____

Appointment date

____

Time

____

5 minute clinic

6 Jokes to Break the Ice with Your Doctor

1. **Patient:** If I take these little green pills just like you say, will I get better?

   Doctor: Well, let's put it this way—none of my patients has ever come back for more pills.

2. **Patient:** Doctor, how can I live to be a hundred?

   Doctor: I suggest you give up eating rich food and going out with women.

   Patient: And then I'll live to be a hundred?

   Doctor: No, but it will seem like it.

3. A seven-year-old girl told her mom, "A boy in my class asked me to play doctor." "Oh no," the mother nervously sighed, "what happened, honey?" "Nothing. He made me wait forty-five minutes and then double-billed Medicare."

4. **Patient:** I keep seeing spots in front of my eyes.

   Nurse: Have you ever seen a doctor?

   Patient: No, just the spots.

5. A man yells into the phone, "My wife is pregnant and her contractions are only two minutes apart!" "Is this her first child?" the doctor asks. "No, you idiot," the man shouts, "this is her husband."

6. A man went to his doctor suffering from a bad cold. His doctor told him to rest, but that didn't help. On the next visit, the doctor gave him some pills, but they didn't help. On the next visit, the doctor gave him a shot, but that didn't help. On the fourth visit, the doctor told the man, "Go home and take a hot bath. After your bath, open all the windows and stand in the cold draft." "But Doctor," the man protested, "if I do that I'll catch pneumonia." "I know," said the doctor. "*That* I can cure."

After Your Visit

Your visit to your doctor doesn't end when you leave the office. If your doctor is doing his job, you will probably have some kind of follow-up: test results to get, a decision to make about treatment, another doctor to see, a treatment plan to follow, or even another appointment to discuss your health further. If you've got a top-notch physician who's completely organized and has a fantastic support staff, you may get a follow-up call, report, or even mailing. But chances are, you are on your own to make sure you follow through.

Before you leave the office you should understand how long the treatment (if you agreed on one) will take to work, what relief in your symptoms you should see, and what side effects you might expect. If what you're experiencing doesn't match what your doctor told you to expect, call the office right away and let them know.

7 Questions to Ask about New Prescriptions

1. Why are you prescribing this medication?
2. How quickly will the drug take effect?
3. What change will I see in my condition?
4. How should I take the medication?
5. What if I miss a dose?
6. What side effects are common?
7. What are the signs of a dangerous reaction?

If you get started on a treatment but find it difficult to stick with, schedule a follow-up appointment to talk about it. For example, if you start experiencing side effects you don't like from a medication your doctor prescribed, don't just stop taking it. Call your doctor to find out if your side effects are normal and will go away. If not, you should let her know you don't want to take it. Often there are other medications or even different therapies to substitute for the drug you're taking. Understand exactly how to take any medications that are prescribed, the possible side effects, and why you are taking it.

RESOURCE

Quick Reference on Medical Tests

Refer to the Appendix for a simple description of the most common medical tests and procedures.

Make sure you show up for any tests your doctor has ordered and you have agreed to. Find out beforehand if the test carries any risks and if there is anything special you need to do to prepare. Talk with your doctor about anxiety you have about the test and ask if there will be any discomfort. Doctors tend to significantly underestimate the physical and mental discomfort of tests, so be sure you understand the value of the test and agree that it's necessary. On the flip side, patients tend to overestimate the discomfort, often working themselves into a state of anxiety. Talking with your doctor beforehand can help you realistically prepare both mentally and physically.

Last, if your doctor has ordered a test, always, always call to get your test results. Don't rely on the doctor to call you. Ask the office staff when you can expect the results and mark your calendar to call them. One study found that 75 percent of physicians did not notify patients of normal test results and 33 percent did not always notify them of abnormal test results. It's estimated that one-third of the women with abnormal mammograms or Pap smears don't receive follow-up care.

Pop Quiz! **Serious Symptoms**

1. A sudden excruciating headache may be a sign of a brain aneurysm. True False
2. A fever accompanied by a stiff neck can be a symptom of a migraine headache. True False
3. Reye's syndrome, a swelling of the brain and liver, can be triggered by giving aspirin to a child. True False
4. Appendicitis is characterized by constant pain in the lower left abdomen. True False
5. A sudden loss of vision in one or both eyes can indicate a stroke. True False

Answers

1. True. Aneurysms can be fatal, so get immediate treatment.
2. False. Migraines are not accompanied by a fever. These symptoms can indicate meningitis.
3. True. Children should never be treated with aspirin.
4. False. Appendicitis pain begins below the belly button and moves to the lower right abdomen. If the pain stops suddenly, it can mean the appendix has burst. Get immediate medical attention.
5. True. Swift treatment is essential to minimizing damage.

Just What Does "Negative" Mean, Anyhow?

Understanding Test Results

Over ten billion medical tests are conducted—forty tests per person—each year in the United States. Tests give doctors and patients valuable information, but often the results are bewildering or scary or some combination of both. Here are some tips for understanding your results:

When Negative Isn't Negative

The terminology used to report test results is confusing to almost everyone. Although we think of *negative* as a bad thing, the term is commonly used in medical testing to indicate the absence of an abnormal condition. Translation: a negative biopsy means that no cancer was found. But obviously doctors also use "negative prognosis" to indicate a condition they believe may have a negative effect on a patient's health. Don't assume—ask your doctor to interpret your test results in a way you understand.

When Positive Doesn't Mean Positive

Unfortunately, no test is absolutely accurate. Mistakes can occur for lots of reasons, including how the test is performed or how the results are read. These mistakes are called false-positives (when the test mistakenly says you have a condition) or false-negatives (when the test misses something that is there). Almost every test has a false-positive rate. For example, the PSA test used to detect prostate cancer in men has recently been determined to have such a high false-positive rate that a debate rages as to whether it works. Many doctors feel that men who receive a false-positive may embark on further invasive tests or treatments with side effects like impotence or incontinence, all for a condition they never had. You should always talk to your doctor about what the rate is for the specific test you're having. And if you get a positive reading, ask to have the test repeated just to be sure.

What Is Normal?

The normal range for most medical tests is set to include only 95 percent of healthy people, so you can get an abnormal result even if you are perfectly healthy. Ask your doctor to interpret the results for you.

Average Isn't Always Good

Right now, average weights, average blood pressure, and average cholesterol rates are all elevated in our population. So make sure when you get your test results that you know what optimum readings are, not just the average. You want to make sure you're going for the gold.

Absolutes Usually Don't Exist

Many tests aren't scientific, appearances to the contrary. Things like MRIs, EKGs, X-rays, and ultrasounds rely on the interpretation of trained experts. Even radiologists admit that you can't really teach someone how to accurately read an X-ray. It's a skill that must be learned by looking at hundreds and hundreds of films. One study determined that 41 percent of chest X-ray readings showed significant errors. Don't be afraid to ask for a second opinion if your test results aren't supported by your symptoms or your condition.

5. What to Expect When You're a Patient

As a patient, you should have certain expectations of your doctors and others giving you care. Remember that the guiding rule for doctors around the world since ancient times has been "first, do no harm." It is my hope that the self-knowledge you've gained from this book gives you the insight to find a doctor who cares, the power to demand the care you deserve, and the skills to build a strong relationship among quality professionals.

Here are some expectations you should have of your doctors and others providing you with care:

- That he will understand and respect who you are as a person, your values, and your health goals.
- That she will explain tests, procedures, and treatments in a way you can understand.
- That you will always be given the most complete, accurate information available on your health and your conditions.
- That she will never coerce or pressure you into a treatment or a therapy.
- That the privacy of your medical information will always be respected.
- That no treatment or information about a treatment will ever be withheld because of financial considerations.
- That he or his staff will respond to your calls or requests within a reasonable amount of time.
- That she will do what she can to help you be as healthy as possible, manage any pain, and live as full a life as you can.

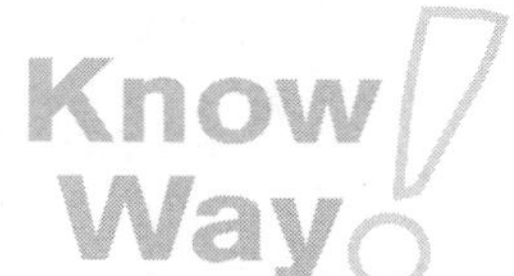

One of the most famous "doctors"—Dr Pepper—was invented by a pharmacist in Waco, Texas, in 1885.

Taylor's Fourth Law of Health

Ignorance is not bliss;
it's just ignorance.

Prescription 3

Know Your Vital Signs

Know Time Like the Present

When most people think about their health, they think about doctors and hospitals. But the path to a healthy life doesn't start at County General—it begins and ends with you. Virtually all of the decisions you make about your health are made away from a doctor's office. Think about the amount of time you spend in a year talking with your doctor . . . for many of us it's nonexistent; for the rest, it's not much more. If you're managing a health condition or getting treatment, you'll see your doctors more, but even then, the percentage of time you spend with them is tiny. Compare that to the number of decisions you make every day about your health—what to eat, when to exercise, what drugs to take, when to get treatment. You really are in charge of your health, whether you realize it or not. The hundreds of decisions you make every day are, by far, the critical factors in your health and well-being. The question is, How prepared are you to make those decisions?

Let's look at something as simple as the medications we take. A

2006 study conducted at the University of California, Los Angeles, found that on average, doctors give patients only 62 percent of the information they need to take their medications correctly. "This is a good indication that there is actually a lack of communication between patients and doctors," says study author Derjung M. Tarn. "And if patients don't get this information from their physician, they might not get it elsewhere since a lot of the information is not included on medication packaging or inserts."

And to add insult to injury (or injury to injury, as the case may be), another study shows that the number of medication errors go up as the number of doctors you use increases. Seniors—the focus of the study—who got prescriptions from two doctors were at risk for ten errors on average; those with five doctors were at risk for sixteen errors. Some of the problems that occur include being prescribed a drug that reacts with another drug you're taking, using a medication that makes another medical condition worse, and getting incorrect dosages and mixed-up medications.

Most of us go almost all the way through life as complete strangers to ourselves.

—SYDNEY J. HARRIS, AUTHOR, *THE AUTHENTIC PERSON*

The Best Candidate for the Job

The bottom line is that you can't depend on anyone or anything else—no doctor, computer, nurse, technician, or pharmacist—to take the care with your health and safety that you will. I discussed earlier in the book the risks you face from medical mistakes, physician error, medication dangers, and risks in the hospital, to name just a few. The dangers from these risks are making the news more and more—1.5 million injuries from medication mistakes, 100,000 people dead from medical mistakes, 1.8 million people who get infections in the hospital—and are at least, in part, able to be measured. What's even more distressing is what I call the "silent killer" that lurks in our health care system—the number of people who get ill or die unnecessarily because their symptoms and conditions went unrecognized, undiagnosed, and untreated until it was too late. A forty-year-old, otherwise healthy woman is diagnosed with end-stage lung cancer and dies four months later. A forty-seven-year-old man drops dead from a heart attack seemingly without any warning. We all have family members, friends, coworkers, and acquaintances who have suffered this fate. For some reason, we're willing to accept these losses as part of the game. Four people killed by anthrax makes the headline news for months. Four hundred thousand people die each year from lung cancer, and it barely merits a mention.

John Kitzhaber, an M.D. and the former governor of Oregon, witnessed firsthand many policy decisions that flew in the face of reason. He tells the tale of one man in his mid-thirties, Douglas Schmidt, who was no longer able to afford his $14-a-day antiseizure medication because of cuts in Medicaid prescription drug benefits. As a result, Douglas suffered a grand mal seizure, ending up with severe brain damage on a ventilator in a Portland hospital. The cost of the intensive care unit was more than $7,500 per day for a total cost of over $1 million. Mr. Schmidt, Dr. Kitzhaber had concluded, died because of policies that will spend millions for care, after the fact, for stroke patients, premature infants, and others who fall victim to conditions that could have been easily prevented for dollars a day. Dr. Kitzhaber gives his take on what has to happen to stop this insanity: "We are running out of time here . . . What we need is a revolution—not of

5 minute clinic

9 Top Ways Patients Sabotage Their Care

Here are some of the top ways we keep ourselves from getting good care and feeling our best.

1. **We don't report all our symptoms.** We often don't tell doctors about all of our symptoms because we're embarrassed, or we think it doesn't matter, or the doctor didn't ask. We also wait to report our symptoms, denying something might be wrong until it's a problem.
2. **We don't provide a list of all medications.** Research suggests that most of us don't report all prescription and over-the-counter medications to our doctors, making it even harder to make sure what they're prescribing is safe.
3. **We don't disclose alternative treatments.** We worry our doctors may get angry or think we're crackpots, but again, this can affect treatments your doctor is prescribing.
4. **We don't follow treatment plans.** Whether out of laziness, financial difficulties, or just not wanting to do it, about 60 percent of us don't follow doctor's orders.
5. **We aren't honest.** We often aren't honest about our symptoms, healthstyle habits, or reasons for choices we make about our health.
6. **We are afraid of our doctors.** We're afraid to tell our doctors we don't want a treatment, don't understand something, or need more information.
7. **We pressure our doctors.** We sometimes pressure our doctors into giving us medications or treatments that may not be in our best interest.
8. **We don't understand.** We often don't take the time to read and follow directions.
9. **We don't take charge.** We sit back and wait for the doctor to take the lead in our health.

violence but of vision; not of arms but of ideas. It is unlikely, however, that the leadership to spark this revolution will come from our political establishment—which means that if we want anything to happen, we will have to make it happen ourselves. It means the responsibility to bring about reform does not belong to someone else. It belongs to us—to you and me."

Is that possible? Can we change our health care system? We may not be able to change the system overnight, but we can change the way we interact with the system—by becoming more empowered, taking charge, and demanding that we get the care we deserve, the care we've paid for. One night I was working late at the office and the phone rang. On the other end I found someone who made me see the difference each one of us can make.

"Are you the people who published this diabetes health organizer book?" the woman on the line asked me.

"Yes," I said, my interest piqued.

"Well, I just wanted to thank you. My name's Elke. I've from New York. I've had diabetes all my life—I'm sixty-two—and this is the first book that ever told me that I need to take care of myself and gave me a way to do it. I'm in a wheelchair and I have to go twelve blocks to my drugstore to get my drugs. Last night I went down there and the man at the pharmacy gave me the wrong pills. I said, 'Look here, son, that's the wrong stuff.' He argued and argued and told me that I was wrong. I didn't have my book with me even though you told me to write down my medicines. But I went back home, got my book, went back down there, and showed him what it was supposed to be. Seems he read the prescription wrong. Well, he apologized up one side and down the other, but I just told him that next time I hoped he would listen up before he killed somebody. He got real quiet and said, 'Yes, ma'am, I will.' That darn book saved my life. I just wanted to let you know."

But Elke was wrong. It wasn't that book that saved her life. It was her—her power, her strength, her persistence, her willingness to take the time and the trouble to save her own life. Did she change that

How to Get the Care You Deserve

You don't have to sit back and accept substandard health care. Here are a few things you can do to make sure you're getting the care you deserve.

- Find out the cost of every health service you use.
- Understand the services and resources your health plan offers and use them to stay healthy.
- Find great doctors and recommend them to your friends and family.
- Ask for clarification when being given a drug, a treatment, or a diagnosis.
- Make sure you understand and agree with instructions and directions. Ask until you do.

Know Way!

According to the *Journal of the American Medical Association*, properly prescribed medications, used properly, are the fourth-leading cause of death in the United States, due to unintended adverse side effects.

young pharmacist? I don't know, but I hope so, even just a little. I do know after talking with her for quite a while that she had a new outlook on her health. Despite how tough it was for her to get good care, how hard she had to work to keep herself feeling well, she knew that no one else was going to do it for her. Her strength and determination were an honor to hear. But it's going to take each one of us, like Elke, to take charge, take the lead, and put our health first. Don't wait for the system to take care of you, because that idea went missing a long time ago. Be responsible for yourself.

Hypertension Harry

Here's an experiment I've tried on over a hundred people who have told me they have high blood pressure. (Considering that an estimated 70 percent of the people with high blood pressure don't even know they have it, just knowing you do puts you ahead of the curve!)

Taylor: So you know a lot about your health?
Harry: Yeah, I have high blood pressure, so I really stay on top of it.
Taylor: So what is your blood pressure?
Harry: I don't know, but I know it's high.
Taylor: How long have you had high blood pressure?
Harry: Not sure, couple of years maybe.
Taylor: Really? Has it gone up in the last couple of years or stayed the same?
Harry: It's gotten better, I think, but it's still pretty high.
Taylor: What's a good blood pressure range for you?
Harry: I'm not sure, but my doctor said if it didn't get better, I would have to start taking blood pressure medicine.

Now, I'm not picking on Harry or his doctor. I was surprised to discover that only about five people out of those I asked had any idea either what their blood pressure reading is or what it should be.

But that's just high blood pressure, right? Surely if you had a "real" disease like diabetes, you'd know how to manage it and take care of yourself. Consider that over 18 million Americans have type 2 (adult onset) diabetes. In a recent poll of people with type 2 diabetes, 98 percent believe that blood sugar control is important to managing their condition. However, 61 percent of those polled weren't aware of the most vital blood sugar test, the A1C, and even after being told what it was, 51 percent didn't know their last A1C result.

It's almost unbelievable that people are walking around with conditions that, while not immediately life-threatening, could shorten their life, and they don't have even basic knowledge about the condition or what to do about it. Many conditions such as type 2 diabetes and heart disease, if discovered early enough, can be treated in a way that's not too disruptive to your life. But the longer you wait to get treatment and manage your condition, the more it will weaken your body and impact your life, becoming harder and harder to treat.

5 Worst Health Inventions

1. Remote control and cable TV
2. Backpack
3. Processed food
4. Escalator
5. Cigarettes

Take Harry, for example. If Harry is twenty-seven when he and his doctor notice that his blood pressure is starting to go up, his condition can be tracked easily enough by using a home blood pressure cuff or even those machines in the grocery store. His doctor could suggest, "Hey, Harry, why don't you try cutting back on salt in your diet?" or "Try adding about thirty minutes more of exercise a week to your routine." For young, strapping, carefree Harry, this is no big deal. He takes up tennis, meets a beautiful young partner at the tennis court, stops salting his french fries so much, and voilá! At his next physical, Harry is happy to report his blood pressure is back in the normal range.

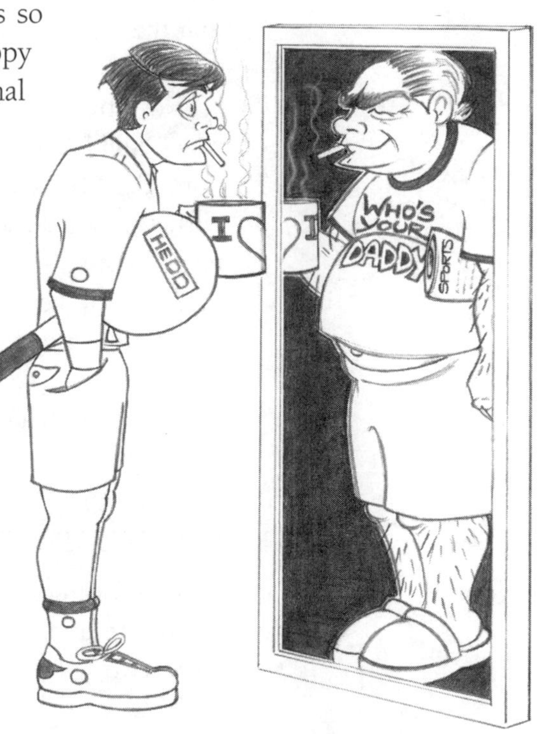

But let's say Harry's fifty-seven. Considerably overweight, with no real exercise routine, he's stressed out at work and at home. "Harry," the doctor says, "I'm really concerned about your blood pressure. It's moving into the dangerous range. I think we need to get you on medication right away to try and bring it down and also make some changes in your diet and exercise." Because of his high blood pressure levels, now Harry's got to take a drug for his hypertension. Some of the side effects Harry experiences include impotence, insomnia, and depression (where's that cute tennis girl now?). Doc wants him to cut out all fried foods and alcohol ("Not beer, too!") and walk for thirty minutes every day. A great idea, but Harry's busy, works too much, and just doesn't have time. The likelihood of Harry being able to incorporate these changes into his life at this age are much slimmer (no pun intended) than if he had started down this road years before.

That's why ignorance is not bliss. Not knowing doesn't make a health condition go away—it only makes it worse when you do have to face it. If you were strapped sitting on top of a suitcase with a ticking bomb and you had in your hand the combination to defuse the bomb, would you defuse it right away, or just sit there and wait until the counter was at thirty seconds? That answer is simple, but so is the answer of understanding your health and taking charge today.

What You Don't Know Can Kill You

In a survey commissioned by CIGNA Healthcare in 2002, 92 percent of those surveyed said it is important to become more informed about their health, with 86 percent saying they should be more actively involved in making health decisions. Yet well over a third also said that they lacked the information or the understanding to make good decisions.

Not knowing your vital information is just—oh, how can I put it?—*Dumb!* I'm not pointing fingers at anyone, or else I'd have to point right back at myself. My daughter, Samantha, got hit in the face with a piñata stick that broke her nose. I showed up at the ER with nothing but a scared five-year-old with blood running down her face and my car keys. As the nurse asked me what sounded like very simple questions—her weight, her last tetanus shot—I responded like most people probably would: "Huh?" Later, I imagined how much worse that could have been if Sam had been in a more serious situation.

One surgeon told me how critical a small bit of information can be to keeping you alive.

> I was doing an operation on a guy—pretty routine, nothing life-threatening. So I got in there and the guy just kept bleeding and bleeding. I looked at the chart and couldn't find anything in his history or chart to tell me what was going on. I asked the prep

nurse over and over if she missed something. Damn, I was pissed—the guy was bleeding out on the table—I was losing him, for no apparent reason. I clamped him off, told the team to keep him stabilized, and went out to talk to his wife. I asked her, "Is there any medication he's taking that he didn't tell us about?"

"No," she told me, "he doesn't take anything—I don't understand."

"Well, I'm going to have to close him back up until we figure this out," I told her.

As I turned to walk back to surgery she nearly whispers, "Well, he does take an aspirin every day for his heart, but that doesn't matter, does it?"

Bingo! It thins the blood—a condition that can kill you during a surgery. That's why aspirin is used as a heart attack treatment. So I go back in and close him up—he's going to have to go off the aspirin for a couple of weeks before we can operate again. Three weeks later we do the surgery—complete success, quick recovery. When I think this guy could have died from an aspirin . . ."

While it might seem trivial, this information is life and death when it comes right down to it. We have at our disposal the best technology and knowledge about health in the history of the planet. Yet millions die and get sick each year who don't have to. Here's some precautions you can take whether at your doctor's office or in the hospital to protect your life and that of those you love.

12 Ways to Save Your Life

1. **Take charge of your health care.** Patients who are more involved in their care are less likely to be the victim of a medical mistake.
2. **When you get a prescription, make sure you can read it.** Ask the doctor to write the purpose of the drug on the prescription so the pharmacist can double-check that he's reading it correctly. Ask your pharmacist to read it back to you so you can check, too. Check the medicine when you pick it up to make sure it's what your doctor prescribed and that the dosage is

RESOURCE

A Handy Way to Record Your Health Information

Download a free health information wallet card at www.tayloryourhealth.com/resources_free_wallet.html.

correct. The state of Massachusetts estimates that 2.4 *million* prescriptions are filled improperly each year there alone.

3. **Tell each of your doctors all of the medications you take.** Include prescriptions, over-the-counter, vitamins, supplements, and herbs.
4. **Be sure you understand new medications.** What is it for? How much do I take? How often do I take it? What food, drink, and activities should I avoid while taking this medication? What would an adverse reaction be and what should I do if that happens?
5. **Always call and get the results for any lab tests you have.** Ask for a written report of your test results and an explanation from your doctor of what they mean. Don't assume "no news is good news."
6. **Find out if your doctor is doing enough.** Check the national guidelines to make sure you're getting at least the minimum recommended treatment. A reliable source for treatment standards can be found from the National Guidelines Clearinghouse at www.guideline.gov.
7. **More isn't always better.** Know why you are having a test, treatment, or new medication prescribed—and what side effects you could have, both long- and short-term. You might decide you would be better off without it.
8. **If you're having surgery, make sure that you, your doctor, and your surgeon are all clear on what is going to be done.** Wrong-site surgery is rare, but don't be afraid to write on your body parts with an indelible marker to let them know where the operation site is and isn't. It's your body, so take it seriously.
9. **Ask who is going to do your surgical procedure.** Doctors often use residents (doctors in training), physician assistants, and other doctors to assist them during surgeries. It's your right to know who will be doing what and their qualifications.
10. **In the hospital, ask anyone you come in contact with to wash their hands.** Although hand-washing is an important way to prevent the spread of infections, it's estimated that only 17 percent of physicians wash their hands as they move between patients.

11. **Before having any procedure, check the background of the person doing the procedure as well as the facility where it will be performed.** Ask the doctor how many times he has performed the procedure. Make sure the hospital you choose has a lot of experience with your procedure.
12. **When you are in the hospital, ask someone close to you to be your advocate.** You may be unconscious, and even if you're wide awake, it pays to have another set of eyes and ears to make sure you understand and approve of what's going on. And if you have a child in the hospital, try to have someone with her as often as possible to make sure her treatments, medications, and care are administered correctly.

> **RESOURCE**
>
> **How Does Your Hospital Rate?**
>
> See how your hospital ranks against others in the nation by clicking on www.qualitycheck.org.

You don't have to be a passive victim of the system. Instead, you can take steps to pull back those covers (c'mon, Chicken Little), pull your head out of the sand (hello, little Ostrich), and find the power to make the system work for you and help you have the long and healthy life you deserve. All twelve of the tips above have one thing in common—taking an active role in your health care. Don't be afraid to offend a health care provider. Their feelings aren't nearly as important as your life, and good professionals will be right there with you demanding the best care.

Isn't There Someone Taking Care of This for Me?

In September 2005, after Hurricane Katrina, lots of stories were told of hurricane victims unable to get AIDS or diabetes medicines, needing treatment or surgery for heart disease, cancer, kidney disease, and all imaginable types of conditions. Yet virtually no one had treatment plans, prescriptions, diagnoses, or even the simplest of health information. This tragedy resulted in a call for physicians and hospitals to transfer health information to computers, called Electronic Medical Records—a ten-year, multibillion-dollar undertaking. But this won't solve the more important issue of how to have this vital information at your fingertips when you need it to save your life and to help you better manage your health.

In an emergency, doctors and hospitals are displaced just like the rest of us. Their records, whether on paper or in a computer, may be, in the worst case, destroyed and in the best case inaccessible for who knows how long. The single best person to keep track of your medical information is *you*. Knowing and keeping track of your vital health information will not only keep you and your family members prepared for any emergency, but will let you begin your journey to take charge of your health. You'll be better prepared for doctor or emergency room visits and better informed when you go to the doctor. You'll understand where your health risks lie and what simple steps you can take to start feeling better and living longer. And you'll be able to give your doctors the information they need to help you prevent health conditions and diagnose and treat conditions before they impact your life and your health.

RESOURCE

Free Medical Record Request

Download a free form you can fax to your doctor to request your records at www.tayloryourhealth.com/free_forms.html.

Your Seven Vital Signs

There are seven key areas or Vital Signs that everyone should know about their health. Don't worry, it's not complicated or hard to do. The great part is that most of this information is right there in your head or easy to find. You've just got to gather any medical records and information you have, organize it, and write it down somewhere so that you, your loved ones, and your doctors can it use to help protect your life and keep you healthy. I'm going to show you exactly how to do that. For each Vital Sign, I'll tell you exactly what you need to know and give you some examples of the kinds of information you'll want to have.

Your 7 Vital Signs

1. The Essential You
2. Your Personal Health Assessment
3. Your Medications
4. Your Health History
5. Your Family Health History
6. Your Doctors
7. Your Health Expenses

Along with the information you're able to remember or gather yourself, you will want to contact doctors or other health professionals you've seen in the past to request your records. Once you've made a list of your doctors, fax each of them a request that includes your name, signature, and where they should send the records. Be sure to ask for records that pertain to their specialty such as Pap smear results from your gynecologist or X-rays from your orthopedist. Some doctors may require a small administration fee or ask that you come and pick up the documents (if you live locally) so that you can sign for them in person. Keep in mind that this is *your* information, so no one should balk at giving you the records.

Records to Request from Your Doctors

Include these in the records you request from each of your doctors:

- List of prescribed medications
- Lab reports (such as bloodwork and cholesterol tests)
- Immunization records
- Your patient file
- Diagnostic tests (such as EKGs, MRIs, biopsies, and mammograms)
- Reports on any surgeries or outpatient procedures you have had

vital sign 1 The Essential You

The Essential You is the basic health information that everyone should have handy at all times. This is the critical information your family members, emergency personnel, and doctors must be able to get their hands on easily when you need care. This information will also give you a good place to start your Healthy Life Plan and move on to your other Vital Signs.

You'll need information about your basic medical condition—things like medical conditions, allergies and medications—as well as the names and numbers of your essential health resources and emergency contacts. But before you get started, let's take a little quiz to find out how much you already know about The Essential You!

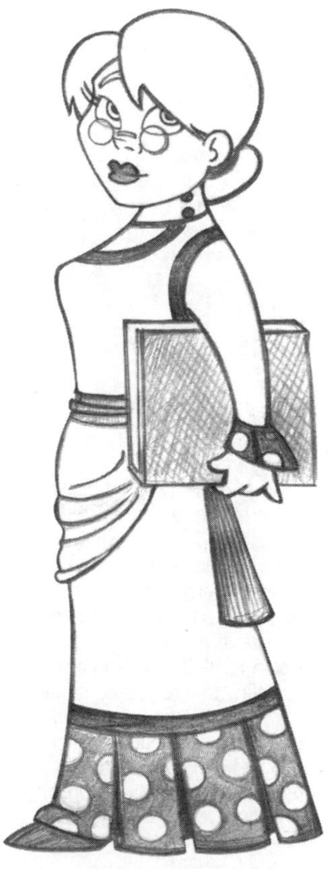

What's Your Health IQ?

How well do you know yourself? Let's see how you rate as an expert on your own health. Take the quiz beginning on page 92 to rate your Health IQ. Without going to any other records or asking anyone else, see how many of the items you can fill in off the top of your head.

Even if your score was in the lower range, you're on the right track. By getting a start on your first Vital Sign, you're well on the road to improving your Health IQ and getting yourself ready to be more prepared when it comes to your health information. The Essential You is the foundation of the information you'll want to gather about your health. And you've taken one of the most important steps you can take in knowing your Vital Signs—you've written them down. It seems like common sense, but very few people have their important health information written down someplace where they and their family members can easily find it. Putting it down on paper is going to be the key to helping you understand your health, be in a position to manage it, and have

What's Your Health IQ?

1. Who are you? (This one's free!)

Name ______________________________________

Address ______________________________________

City ____________________ State __________ Zip ____________

Phone __________________ e-mail ____________________

2. The basics

Sex: ☐ Male ☐ Female

Date of birth ______________________________________

Social Security number ______________________________

3. What's your weight?

Pounds __________________ Kilograms* __________________

4. What's your height?

Feet __________________ Inches __________________

5. What's your blood type? (Check one of each.)

Blood type: ☐ A ☐ B ☐ AB ☐ O

RH factor: ☐ positive ☐ negative

6. What medical conditions do you have?

____

____

7. What allergies do you have?

____

____

*Why should I know my weight in kilograms?

Kilograms is used by health care professionals to calculate medication dosages. Knowing your weight in kilograms is useful in an emergency situation so that you aren't relying on someone else to do the weight conversion for you. It is especially important to know this about your children, since even small fluctuations can mean the difference between an appropriate dose and a dangerous overdose.

To find your weight in kilograms, just divide your weight in pounds by 2.2.

What's Your Health IQ?

8. Who is your doctor?

Name ____________________

Address ____________________

Phone ____________ e-mail ____________

9. What is your health insurance information?

Company ____________________

Subscriber ____________________

Policy No. ____________________

Group No. ____________________

Phone ____________ e-mail ____________

10. Who is your emergency contact?

Name ____________________

Address ____________________

Phone ____________ e-mail ____________

11. What drugs have you taken in the last six months?

____

____

12. Where is your Living Will?

____

13. Who is your Durable Power of Attorney designee?

Name ____________________

Address ____________________

Phone ____________ e-mail ____________

What's your score?

Give yourself a point for each question you answered correctly.

11–13 correct
Healthificacious!
Ready for emergencies and staying on top of your health.

7–10 correct
Health Conscious
Good start on becoming healthy—keep going.

4–6 correct
Health Unconscious
Having an out-of-body experience.

0–3
Health Oblivious
Closing your eyes and hoping for the best?

Keeping Your Private Info Private

Nearly 70 percent of Americans are concerned about the privacy of their health information. Here are a few precautions you can take to help protect your health and your privacy.

- Don't put it online.
- Don't sign any blanket releases.
- Ask your doctor who has access to your info.
- Don't give it out over the phone or in surveys.

a record that you can use to help doctors give you the right care and make the right treatment decisions when your life is at stake. You can make a copy of these pages and keep it handy so you have instant access to your important information anytime.

You need information that can speak for you if you can't. Even if you scored an astounding 13 and are one of the rare people who know all of these facts off the top of your head, consider for a moment that you've just been in a car collision. You may be disoriented or even unconscious. You may be so shaken up you can't remember your own name, let alone your doctor's. And if you're not able to communicate for yourself, this information will help family members get you treatment instead of standing by and feeling helpless. Be sure that you give a copy of the above information to the person who is your emergency contact as well as other family members or friends. The information won't do you any good if nobody knows where to find it when it's needed.

A Living Will describes what level of care you would want in case you are unable to speak for yourself. A Durable Power of Attorney for Health Care gives someone close to you the authority to make decisions about your health if you cannot. Both these advance directives can be important in making decisions about your care.

vital sign 2 Your Personal Health Assessment

Now that you've got the essentials down, it's time to gather information on your everyday health. Your Personal Health Assessment will help you evaluate your healthstyle, highlight some areas where you might be at risk, and set the stage for you to develop your Healthy Life Plan.

The Personal Health Assessment isn't going to assess your risk of diabetes or tell you that you're at risk for lung cancer because you smoke. It's going to help you think about seven important areas of your health and highlight where you can make changes to feel better and live longer within those seven areas. It doesn't mean that there aren't other things you can do or that you don't have other risks. The Personal Health Assessment is just a way for you to start taking charge of your health and help you see that your doctor can do more for you if you start doing more for yourself.

The Personal Health Assessment will also give you a great tool you can use to start talking with your doctor about what you can do to improve your health. Many times a patient will say, "I want to be healthier," without giving specifics on what they want to improve. The Personal Health Assessment will help you and your doctor pinpoint reasonable actions you can start taking right away. You'll also see small things you can do, like wearing a seat belt, using sunscreen, and checking your smoke detectors, that can make a big difference in your health and safety.

After you take the Personal Health Assessment, you're going to use it to build a Healthy Life Plan that will let you find the health power to stay healthy, feel better, and live longer.

Lifestyle Habits Evaluation

If any of your answers here indicate a risk, you'll want to take a look at the lifestyle choices you make to see where you can begin a plan to improve your health. Keep in mind that these four lifestyle choices can affect people in any age group, any economic group, and all ethnicities. Because these are lifestyle choices that we make, none of us are immune to their effects. For example, many people think that risky sexual behaviors occur only in the young or that people who abuse drugs are in a low socioeconomic group. That's simply not true.

For example, the availability of drugs to treat erectile dysfunction has led to an increase in sexually transmitted diseases in people over age sixty. Often mistakenly believing that their risk is lower, many older adults don't take necessary precautions to prevent diseases such as HPV, herpes, and even HIV. One doctor in a central Florida senior active living community says that she has seen a higher incidence of STDs in this small community than when she was a practicing gynecologist in Miami.

Likewise, stereotypes persist about people who might have problems with the use of drugs in their lives. Drug abuse is no longer limited to drugs obtained off the streets like heroin, cocaine, or marijuana. Most patients take medicine responsibly, but according to the National Institute on Drug Abuse (NIDA), 48 million people—representing 20 percent of the U.S. population—have used prescription drugs for a nonmedical purpose in their lifetime. The Food and

Personal Health Assessment

Take the Personal Health Assessment to see how you can lower your risk for conditions and improve your health and safety. A YES or NO in **bold** may show a potential health risk for you, so you'll want to discuss those areas with your doctor and use the Healthy Life Plan in the next chapter to help you come up with ways to minimize those risks.

Lifestyle Habits

Do you **smoke cigarettes**?	☐ **YES**	☐ NO
Do you **chew tobacco**?	☐ **YES**	☐ NO
Do you use **drugs recreationally**?	☐ **YES**	☐ NO
Do you practice **safe sex**?	☐ YES	☐ **NO**
Do you drink more than **four beers**, **four glasses of wine**, or **two cocktails a week**?	☐ **YES**	☐ NO

Healthy Habits

Do you get **physical activity** at least three times a week?	☐ YES	☐ **NO**
Do you **avoid the sun** or wear sunscreen?	☐ YES	☐ **NO**
Do you **brush and floss teeth daily** and have regular dental checkups?	☐ YES	☐ **NO**
Do you **drive safely and wear a seat belt**?	☐ YES	☐ **NO**
Do you have **working smoke detectors** in your home?	☐ YES	☐ **NO**
Do you and your spouse or partner ever have **arguments that result in physical fighting**?	☐ **YES**	☐ NO

Prevention

Do you have a **regular doctor**?	☐ YES	☐ **NO**
Do you have **regular physical checkups**?	☐ YES	☐ **NO**
Are you up to date on **immunizations**?	☐ YES	☐ **NO**
Are you up to date on **preventive screenings**?	☐ YES	☐ **NO**
Do any family members have a **history of diabetes**?	☐ **YES**	☐ NO
Do any family members have a **history of heart disease** or **heart attack**?	☐ **YES**	☐ NO
Do any family members have a **history of cancer**?	☐ **YES**	☐ NO

Self-Care

Women: Do you perform monthly **breast self-exams**?	☐ YES	☐ **NO**
Men: Do you perform monthly **testicular self-exams**?	☐ YES	☐ **NO**

Personal Health Assessment

Cardiovascular Health

My **blood pressure** should be below: ______ / ______

My last reading was: ______ / ______

My healthy **weight** is about: ______

My current weight is about: ______

My **cholesterol** should be: HDL ______ / LDL ______

My last reading was: HDL ______ / LDL ______

Mental Health

Do you **cope well with stress** or seek counseling for problems that become overwhelming?	☐ YES	☐ **NO**
Do you ever have **thoughts of suicide**?	☐ **YES**	☐ NO
Do you often have **feelings of sadness or hopelessness**?	☐ **YES**	☐ NO
Do you ever experience **attacks of panic** or **overwhelming anxiety**?	☐ **YES**	☐ NO
Do you have **interest in daily activities**?	☐ YES	☐ **NO**
Do you have **sleep problems**? (too little or too much)	☐ **YES**	☐ NO

Diet and Nutrition

Do you eat a **variety of nutritious foods**?	☐ YES	☐ **NO**
Do you eat at least **5 to 7 servings of fruits and vegetables** each day?	☐ YES	☐ **NO**
Do you include **grains and fiber** in your diet?	☐ YES	☐ **NO**
Do you eat a lot of **fast foods and frozen meals**?	☐ **YES**	☐ NO
Do you eat a lot of **salty foods** or add salt to your food?	☐ **YES**	☐ NO
Do you eat a lot of foods **high in sugar**?	☐ **YES**	☐ NO
Women: Do you include enough **calcium** in your diet?	☐ YES	☐ **NO**

Drug Administration stresses that prescription drug abuse isn't about bad drugs or even bad people. It involves a complex web of factors, including the power of addiction, misperceptions about drug abuse, and the difficulty both patients and doctors have discussing and understanding the risks of medication abuse.

If You Have Lifestyle Habit Risks

- Have an honest conversation with a doctor who can give you an assessment of how much you are putting your health at risk.
- Determine if there are some simple things you can do to lower your risks (for example, safer sexual practices, cutting back on alcohol, developing a stop-smoking plan, managing your medications better).

Healthy Habits Evaluation

These are the everyday habits where we could all do more to be healthier. While these habits may seem small, the impact they can have on your health can be monumental. For example, over a million people are diagnosed each year with skin cancer. But while skin cancer is the most deadly form of cancer, it is also the most preventable and the most curable. And don't discount the importance of safety in your daily health habits. Despite improved safety features, automobile accidents are still one of the leading causes of death in the United States.

If You Have Healthy Habit Risks

- An easy way to become more physically active is to find things you can include in your daily routine—parking your car at the far end of the lot, taking the stairs whenever possible, walking to school, and so on.

5 minute clinic

5 Ways to Check for Skin Cancer

1. Make a "mole map"—a simple drawing or photograph that shows where the moles are on your body. Research shows that people who map the markings on their body are better able to catch new growths.
2. Ask someone to use a hand mirror to check your back for any changes or suspicious-looking spots. Check your neck, shoulders, arms, lower back, and buttocks.
3. Use a blow-dryer to check your scalp.
4. Sit down to check your legs and feet. Don't forget the soles of your feet and heels.
5. Look for the ABCDE's of skin cancer:
   - **A**symmetry The mole is oddly shaped—one half is different from the other
   - **B**order Ragged or irregular edges
   - **C**olor Varied color: brown, black, blue, white, or red, with a mottled look
   - **D**iameter Bigger than a pencil eraser or increases in size.
   - **E**volving Any changes or symptoms like bleeding

- Use the checklist on page 98 to look at your skin on a regular basis and make sure you take precautions each day to avoid too much sun.
- Improving your driving habits and style is a simple way to make strides in both your physical and mental health. Wearing your seat belt every time you get into a car (and making sure everyone else does, as well) can lower your risk of death or serious injury by 50 percent.
- Aggressive driving not only puts you and others on the road at risk, but raises your blood pressure and places stress on your heart and your mind. Take a deep breath when you get behind the wheel and let go of your anger.
- Make brushing and flossing a daily ritual and get regular checkups at the dentist.
- Perform a safety check on your home every six months to look for and correct any hazards.
- Work on a positive, nurturing relationship with your partner or spouse. Seek counseling either together or separately to address any anger in your relationship.

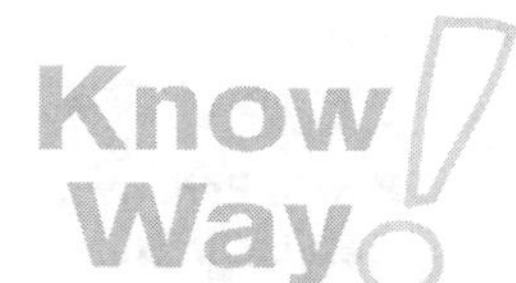

Brushing your teeth before breakfast decreases your chance for cavities. Bacteria in your mouth interact with bacteria on food and add to tooth decay.

Prevention Evaluation

No saying is probably more true when it comes to your health than "A pound of prevention is worth an ounce of cure." In the United States, we are experts at spending thousands to cure something that takes pennies to prevent. This goes for your time as well as your money. Many of us put off having physicals, getting screenings, or getting up to date on immunizations because we just don't have the time. A friend of mine, Tom, told me how his perceptions came crashing to Earth when he was diagnosed with a health condition.

> You know me. I was an eight-days-a-week, twenty-eight-hours-a-day full-blown workaholic. It was go, go, go all the time. I love that saying "Live hard and leave a good-looking corpse." That's all funny when you're saying it, but when it becomes a reality, it's just not as cute. About a year ago I started getting chest pains when I was playing basketball after work. I'm in good shape, so I figured it would go away. But it didn't. Finally my wife nagged me into going to the doctor. I didn't want to. I hadn't had a checkup in about ten years and I knew it was just

RESOURCE

Home Safety Check

You can find safety info on everything from BBQ grills to electrical wiring to appliances and more at www.homesafetycouncil.org.

going to be a bunch of useless tests and a lot of scolding me about taking better care of myself. Not only did I not want to hear it, but I really didn't have the time for this stuff. Well, you know the drill, long story short, it wound up that I had blockages in my arteries and my blood pressure was through the roof, not to mention I've got a family history of early heart disease. Not only did the doctor want me to slow down in general, but man, talk about time-consuming. It seems like every week I have a different test or appointment to keep. Take this medication—wait, that's not working—try this one. Things would have been a lot easier if I had been going to the doctor for checkups and taking better care of myself all along. On the good side, though, it really woke me up to how important it is to worry about my health now. I had this vision of my kids growing up without me—in some ways they already have been—and I decided to put things in a little better perspective."

RESOURCE

How to Perform a Testicular Exam

Download the instructions on performing an exam at www.tayloryourhealth.com/resources_main.html.

If you answered "no" to having a regular doctor or getting regular checkups, you are neglecting one of the most important parts of your preventive care. Regular meetings with a doctor who understands your health will help you stay on top of health risks, get the screenings that you need, and catch any problems as early as possible.

RESOURCE

How to Perform a Breast Exam

Download free instructions on performing an exam at www.tayloryourhealth.com/resources_main.html.

Self-care tests for men and women are also part of the prevention section, including monthly tests for breast and testicular cancer. If you aren't doing monthly self-tests, you're cheating yourself of a valuable early detection tool. You can't always feel a lump, but taking a few minutes a month to check yourself out will certainly be well worth your time if you do find something early.

If You Have Prevention Risks

- Make an appointment *today* for an annual checkup.
- At your checkup, ask your doctor what screenings you might need based on your health, lifestyle choices, and health and family history.
- Ask your doctor if there are any new immunizations that you might be missing.
- Circle a date on your calendar to do your breast or testicular self-exams each month.

Cardiovascular Health Evaluation

Heart disease is the leading killer of adults in this country. The irony is that it's also one of the most easily avoidable. There's a large misconception that places a greater importance on inherited heart conditions than on the lifestyle choices we make. That's just not true. As you can see, the 9 Leading Causes of Heart Attacks are things you can control primarily through your healthstyle choices. Monitoring your vital cardiovascular stats and getting them within a healthy range is an important part of staying on top of your cardio health.

> **5 minute clinic** **9 Leading Causes of Heart Attacks**
>
> Heart disease remains America's number-one killer, claiming more lives than the other top causes combined. Heart disease is responsible for the death of one in five women and over 400,000 men each year.
>
> According to a landmark INTERHEART study encompassing 30,000 men and women in fifty-two countries, there are nine lifestyle factors that are responsible for virtually all the risk for heart attacks. The good news is that all nine factors can be minimized by making simple adjustments in your life, in effect significantly lowering your risk.
>
> 1. Unhealthy weight
> 2. Lack of physical activity
> 3. Smoking
> 4. Unhealthy diet
> 5. Too much alcohol
> 6. High blood pressure
> 7. High cholesterol
> 8. Diabetes
> 9. Emotional issues (such as stress or depression)

If You Have Cardiovascular Health Risks

- Buy a home blood pressure monitor. They're fairly inexpensive and accurate. Knowing your numbers and monitoring your blood pressure over a period of time is the best way to see any upward trends.
- Throw out all your fad diet books and plans and get started on a sensible diet plan that will help you lose weight and keep it off. Ask your doctor what he recommends or if he has a plan he can give you. It should be based around eating a variety of nutritious foods, limiting your calories, and writing down what you eat. These are the proven elements of a successful weight-loss program.

Mental Health Risk Evaluation

Though often ignored at doctor's appointments or in general health advice, the link between your mental health and your physical health simply cannot be denied. There are experts who believe that 90 percent of all health conditions are caused or complicated by stress. And even if you're in perfect physical health, mental health issues cannot only shorten you life, but certainly make life less enjoyable for you as

By the Numbers

How do your numbers compare to these ranges considered healthy?

- Blood pressure—under 120/80
- Total cholesterol—less than 200 mg/dL
- LDL cholesterol (bad)—under 130
- HDL cholesterol (good)—over 45
- At-rest heart rate—60 to 80 beats per minute

well as those around you. As you can see from your Personal Health Assessment, mental health issues can come in many forms, including stress that's overwhelming, panic attacks, and anxiety. Everyone experiences anxiety, sadness, panic, and all kinds of emotions during the course of their day. But if your feelings are interfering with your ability to do your normal activities, causing you sleeping, eating, or other health problems; or are simply overwhelming, you should talk with your doctor or a counselor. Remember that getting help to keep you emotionally well is a sign of strength, not weakness. Panic and anxiety are common emotions and can be a normal reaction to stress or an uncomfortable situation. But if you answered "yes" to having attacks of panic or overwhelming anxiety, these emotions may be putting your mental health at risk. The chart on page 103 will help you determine if your feelings are a passing moment of anxiety or regularly occurring attacks of panic.

Sleep problems, while often related to physical conditions, can also be a sign that your emotions are overwhelming you. Everyone loses sleep now and then, but if you are sleeping either too much or not enough, you should talk with your doctor about possible causes.

RESOURCE

Mental Health Resources, Quizzes, and Forums

Great Web site with info on mental wellness, treatments, and latest news at www.psychcentral.com.

If You Have Mental Health Risks

- If any of these areas were a risk for you, consider finding a counselor, a social worker, or another person you can talk to. You may be able to resolve your problems on your own, but it never hurts to have someone else's perspective on an issue.
- If your emotional issues are disrupting your life, causing problems in your personal relationships or at work, or otherwise keeping you from living a full life, find a way to get help. Taking that first step is often the hardest part, and it helps to know you're not alone.

Diet and Nutrition Risk Evaluation

You know how important the foods you eat every day are to your overall health. This section helps you pinpoint where you might be sabotaging your efforts to improve what you eat. The plain fact is that most Americans do not eat enough fruits and vegetables in their diets.

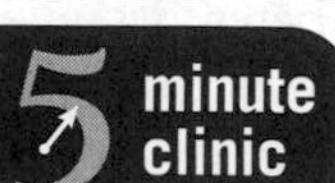

Is It a Panic Attack?

A panic attack can begin suddenly and usually lasts anywhere from thirty minutes to up to a day. You often feel tired and worn out after the attack subsides. Here are some of the more common signs:

- Rapid heartbeat
- Sweating
- Trembling or shaking
- Difficulty swallowing or lump in throat
- Shortness of breath
- Hyperventilation (breathing in and out too fast)
- Feeling light-headed or dizzy
- Chills or hot flashes
- Upset stomach or abdominal cramps
- Chest pain
- Skin losing color
- Having an unreal sense of being in a dream
- A sense of doom
- A feeling that you might die

Many scientists believe that panic attacks are related to your body's normal fight-or-flight instincts. When you are in a situation that your mind perceives as dangerous (such as facing an alligator in the wild), your body will naturally increase your heart rate and you will feel an adrenaline rush to prepare your body either to fight for your life or to flee. When you experience a panic attack, your body responds in the same way, but without being exposed to true danger.

If you often have panic attacks or the fear of an attack keeps you from doing your normal activities or things you enjoy, talk to your doctor about what treatments are available, including talk therapy, cognitive behavioral therapy (see mental health therapies in the Appendix), and medications.

If you answered "no" to five to seven servings, you are in this category. The power these foods have in strengthening your immune system and preventing cancer and heart disease and many other health conditions is nothing short of amazing. If you do nothing else in your diet, make a concerted effort to eat as many fruits and vegetables on a daily basis as you can.

For women of all ages, it's important to include calcium in your diet, so if you answered "no" here, you'll want to look for some good sources. You don't have to pile on the calories to get your calcium—there's lots of good sources, such as broccoli, calcium-fortified orange juice, and fruit-flavored yogurt, in addition to the traditional sources like milk and cheese.

If You Have Diet and Nutrition Risks

- Ask your doctor to recommend a nutritionist you can talk with about a healthy eating plan. Some health insurance plans will cover this service, since it helps you ward off other health problems.

RESOURCE

No-Nonsense Nutrition Guide

A great resource on how to read food labels, lose weight, and eat smart every day is *Smart Guide to Getting Thin and Healthy* by K. Colton.

- If you're managing a health condition like diabetes, it's even more critical to have a sound diet and eating plan to keep your body functioning at its peak.
- Try writing down what you eat over the course of a week to see where you could be missing essential vitamins, minerals, and food groups.

vital sign 3 Your Medications

No one will disagree that in the past fifty years, we have reaped incredible benefits from the development of an enormous range of prescription and over-the-counter drugs. From powerful antibiotics to miraculous heart drugs, from medications to treat once-thought-incurable emotional conditions like depression or obsessive-compulsive disorder to immunizations that have kept millions of children from dying or contracting debilitating diseases like polio, rubella, and meningitis, lives have been lengthened and made healthier by the thousands of drugs we now have access to.

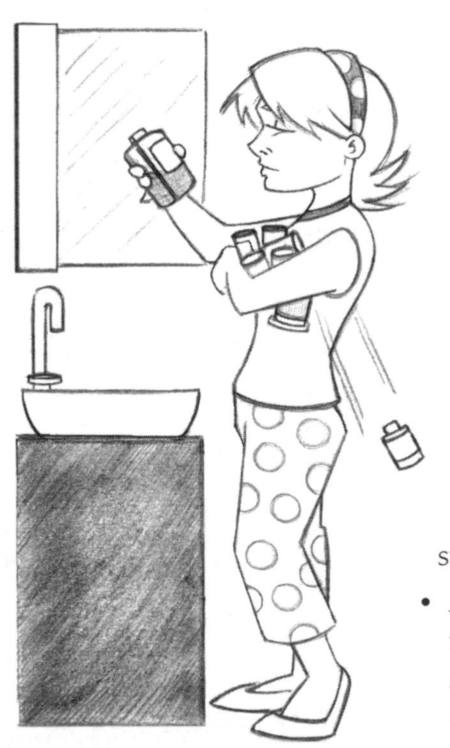

But everything you put in your body, from food to medications to herbs, will affect your body in different ways—some good, some bad. You've got to consider how each drug you take might be affected by, or interact with, other things you take like food, drugs, alcohol, and vitamins. Are adverse reactions and interactions to drugs common? Some experts put the figure as high as 5 million adverse drug reactions each year, although it's difficult to estimate, since only a small percentage are actually reported. At that rate, you're talking about 13,000 incidents each day! In fact, one of every eight people who walk into an ER are having a reaction to something they took—presumably to make them feel better. But adverse reactions aren't the only danger from the drugs we take. Consider these cases:

- An elderly patient with rheumatoid arthritis dies after receiving a 10-milligram *daily* dose of the drug methotrexate, rather than the recommended 10-milligram *weekly* dose.

- A patient with diabetes dies from being given 200 units of insulin rather than the intended 20 units when a dosage was read as "200" rather than "20 U."
- Upon taking her father to the local emergency room for severe back pain, a nurse informs the ER staff that her father had a previous reaction to narcotics and that he shouldn't be given any such drugs. The first night her father is in the hospital (admitted after a 13-hour wait in the emergency room), the neurosurgeon on duty writes a prescription for a morphine patch.
- Premature babies at a hospital in Indiana receive an adult dose of the blood thinner heparin—one thousand times stronger than the dose they should have received. The medicine had been put into the wrong cabinet by a pharmacy technician, a mistake that went unnoticed by the nurses administering the medication. Two of the infants died within hours, and a third died within four days. Crushingly, medical experts say this scenario, rather than being an out-of-the-blue circumstance, is "depressingly normal."
- Two infants in Illinois die after taking cough medication prescribed by their doctors that, while legally sold and widely prescribed by pediatricians, contained a substance not approved by the FDA—the antihistamine carbinoxamine. These drugs are part of the over two thousand unapproved prescription drugs still on the market that were in use before a 1962 amendment required that drugs be approved by the FDA.

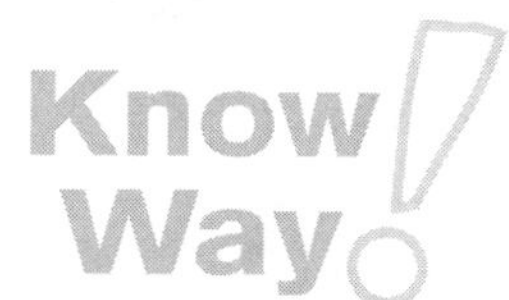

Deaths from medication errors go up 25 percent in the first days of the month because pharmacists are busier and make more mistakes.

These scenarios aren't one-shot mistakes and they make achingly clear a major problem in our health care system. A recent report gives a conservative estimate that 1.5 million people suffer injury each year as a result of medication mistakes. Medication errors and adverse drug reactions like these are medical issues that no one likes to discuss. But in order to do what's needed to fix these problems, we must bring the issue out into the open, talk about it, and learn what we can each do to keep ourselves and our loved ones safe.

In many ways, this problem is another result of how health care technology has developed at a faster rate than our health care system's ability to handle it. When you were a child, how many medications do you remember your grandparents or great-grandparents taking? One, maybe two? The average American takes an estimated ten

RESOURCE

National Poison Control Hotline

Call 9-1-1 or 800-222-1222 if you suspect an adverse drug reaction.

prescription drugs every year. For example, my children see their grandmother take twelve pills a day. And I'm not talking about vitamins or aspirin, but powerful stuff—blood thinners, cancer drugs, cholesterol medication, and so on. These drugs have enabled her to manage her health conditions and live a long, full life that wouldn't have been possible fifty years ago. But an accident that occurred in our lives several years ago demonstrated the seriousness with which these miracle drugs must be handled.

A Flash before My Eyes

My mother had recently returned from (successful!) chemotherapy treatment for breast cancer in Texas. Not having seen her grandchildren in quite a while, she asked if she could pick them up from school and watch them at my house for the afternoon. Knowing that her treatment had really taken it out of her, I asked her several times if she was up to chasing around two small kids. Since my dad would be with her, she assured me she was up to the task. Then came the phone call at work every parent dreads. "Taylor," she said, her voice trembling, "we have a problem."

"What is it?" I asked, already nearly hysterical.

"I think Jack took some of my medicine—no, I know he did. I had it in a case in a drawer and I was taking a nap and I guess he came in and got the case and took it . . ."

"What medication was it?" my voice getting more strained. I held the phone away and screamed for my husband in the next office, "John—Jack's taken Mom's medicine—we're not sure which ones." By now I was in a full-blown panic. There is nothing worse than knowing your child is in danger and you're not there beside him.

John, always the clear thinker, ran into my office and grabbed the phone. "Call 9-1-1 *now*. We're on our way," he said, dragging me out to the car.

It's about a twenty-minute ride from our office to our house, a drive that I think John covered in about ten minutes, although it seemed like an hour. People talk of seeing their life flash before their eyes in a life-and-death situation. I now understood what they meant. During that car ride, I had this crystal-clear vision of sitting at Jack's funeral. I could see the coffin, I could see the stitching on the black dress I was wearing. It wasn't just my imagination, it was almost as if I were seeing it in my memory—as if it had already occurred. I knew at that moment that this little mistake had the potential to impact forever the lives of everyone I loved—Jack, his sister Sam, John, myself, my parents.

We pulled into the driveway—I don't even remember getting out of the car. When I ran into the house I do remember running smack-dab into three very tall, very burly EMTs. But no sign of Jack. "Where's my son?" I asked, fearing the worst.

"Your mother has him in the bedroom, ma'am, and he won't come out. He's scared. But we need to see him right away."

I ran to the bedroom, and there he was. Scared, yes, but he seemed okay. I took him in my arms and ran into the bathroom with him. "Honey," I calmly said, "you're not in any trouble. You didn't do anything wrong. Just tell me if you took Grandma's medicine. It's really important."

I'll never forget the poor little guilty look in his eyes as he nodded "yes." "Okay, what did you take?" I asked, my heart beating in my ears.

"Well," he said in that precious little voice, "I put three in my mouth, but I spit them out because they tasted bad. I thought it was candy."

I think my heart just skipped a beat. "Can you show me where you spit them out?"

5 minute clinic

4 Things to Do If You Think a Child Has Been Poisoned

1. Stay calm and act quickly.
2. Get help immediately if your child has
   - Severe throat pain
   - Excessive drooling
   - Difficulty breathing
   - Convulsions
   - Excessive drowsiness

   Call 9-1-1 or have someone drive you to the closest emergency room.
3. Find what they took.

   If your child has anything remaining in her mouth, make her spit it out or remove it with your finger. Find the container and any remaining contents.
4. Call Poison Control.

   The national hotline is 1-800-222-1222.

   Be ready to tell Poison Control:
   - Your name and phone number
   - Your child's name, age, and weight
   - Any medical conditions the child has
   - Any medications your child takes
   - The name of what she took
   - The time it was taken

Do not make your child throw up unless instructed to do so by Poison Control.

"Okay." Jack then directed me to a bathroom, where I saw two little pills in the garbage can.

"Where's the third one, honey?" As he showed me the last pill in another garbage can, I knew that we had dodged a bullet. I showed the paramedics the pills, and we all breathed a sigh of relief.

"It happens more than you know, ma'am," the paramedics told me, but somehow I wasn't reassured.

RESOURCE

Check before You Take a Drug

Find a free drug interaction checker at www.drugdigest.org.

What I knew, what had engulfed me on that terrible car ride home, was that if something had happened to him, there was only one person to blame. Me. You see, this wasn't the first time my mom had left her medication in a place where the kids could reach it. She and my dad lived alone and they didn't think twice about leaving medication out on the counter. They didn't have to. They, like many older folks, didn't like to have to open the child-resistant containers, so they transferred their medications to little plastic snap-open containers, which to a child look a lot like something that holds candy. I had chastised my mom several times for setting her pill container down on my counter, even finding it once after it had fallen out of her pocket on the family room floor. But I was still the "kid" and could only "correct" my mom so much.

Even worse, when the paramedics arrived, nobody had a detailed list of which medications Jack had put into his mouth. My mom was taking powerful stuff, as I mentioned—blood thinners, heart medication, postchemotherapy treatments—things that pose a real danger to a small child. She knew generally what they were, but couldn't supply either Poison Control or the EMTs with the names and dosages that would have helped save Jack's life, if necessary. We were all humbled by this event and needless to say, my mom felt terrible. But I was determined that I would turn this into a learning experience for us all and for everyone I could tell. I know that I'm one of the lucky ones because Jack suffered no lasting effects. But I also know that incidents like these and harmful reactions to medications or deadly medication mistakes happen every single day and take the lives and the health of people we love.

The Top 10 Medication Mistakes

Listed below are the top causes of medication mistakes and adverse reactions.

1. Wrong drug was prescribed by doctor.
2. Wrong dosage of correct drug was prescribed by doctor.
3. Wrong medication was given to the patient by pharmacist or nurse.
4. Pharmacist read prescription incorrectly.
5. Drug was given where there was a previous allergic reaction. (Sometimes doctors don't check, and sometimes patients don't tell.)
6. Adverse reaction occurs where no previous allergy was known.
7. Drug was given to wrong patient (primarily in hospitals).
8. Wrong dose or wrong mixture was prepared.
9. Drug was given that interacts with another medication used by patient.
10. Wrong drug or dose was taken by patient.

Who's Minding the Drugstore?

At the rate we use medications, the chance for accidental poisonings, dosing mistakes, taking the wrong medication, or taking a medication that reacts with something else increases exponentially. Along with access to all of these drugs comes a lot of responsibility: the responsibility to know what you are putting into your body and to make sure you need it; to safeguard the medications you use so that children or other adults don't take them by mistake; to make sure that it's the right drug in the right amount; to realize that every substance you put into your body affects it in some way, good or bad; to understand how your body will react and how the medication will react with other medications, food, drink, exercise, and so on; to know what to do if you have an adverse reaction. And that's just with prescription drugs. Drugstores today have more drugs available on their shelves for anyone to buy than doctors had in their entire arsenal fifty years ago. We all have a personal chemistry set right in our medicine cabinets, but no training to be sure we don't blow ourselves up!

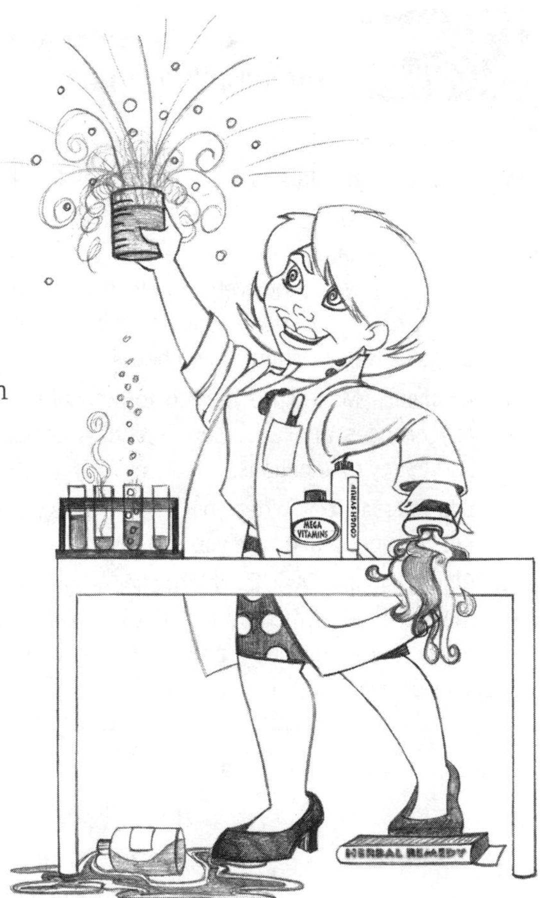

While many pharmacies have sophisticated tracking systems, most of us shop around and use more than one pharmacy. And like any computer system, there's always a chance for unavoidable mistakes—you may be in the same computer system three times, once as Tom E. Jones, once as Tom Jones, and once as Tom Edward Jones, with no link between your three prescriptions. Your doctors should keep track of the medications they've prescribed to you, but they have no way of knowing about over-the-counter drugs you take or drugs prescribed to you by other physicians.

As with most other facets of your health, the best—strike that—the *only* candidate for the job is you. Keeping a detailed list of the medications you take will not only help you avoid mistakes, be ready for emergencies, and understand what you're taking, but will let you review your medications on a regular basis to evaluate with your doctor whether you still need them or if there's anything new that might be more effective for your condition.

5 minute clinic

8 Ways to Be Safer with Prescription Drugs

Here are some of the best ways to make sure that you take the right drug at the right time and in the right amount, right?

1. **Spill the beans.** Make sure that all of your doctors know about everything you are taking, including prescription and over-the-counter drugs as well as vitamins and herbs.
2. **Ah-choo!** Make sure your doctor knows about any allergies and adverse reactions you have had to any medications.
3. **Can *you* read it?** When your doctor writes you a prescription, make sure you can read it.
4. **Plain English.** Ask for information about your medicines in terms you can understand, both when your medicines are prescribed and when your pharmacist gives them to you.
5. **Double check ✓✓** When you pick up your medicine from the pharmacy, ask whether it is the medicine that your doctor prescribed.
6. **Crystal clear.** Before you take any medications, make sure you understand all of the directions about how much to take, when to take it, and what adverse reactions to look for.
7. **Size matters.** Ask your pharmacist what would be the best measuring device if you have liquid medication. A household teaspoon is not the same as a measured teaspoon.
8. **Everybody shout.** Don't be afraid to speak up. If anything isn't clear or if the side effects seem too severe, talk it through with your doctor. Sometimes there are alternate therapies or medications that might be better suited to your individual needs.

If you have any questions or concerns about a drug you are taking, don't hesitate to ask your pharmacist or doctor. And if you've had a reaction or side effect that you think could be related to a medication, tell your doctor immediately and find out what you should do. If you decide to stop taking a medication because of the side effects, tell your doctor this, too. People react differently to medications, and there is usually more than one option for treatment. The doctor may be able to prescribe a different drug that may be effective without the side effect. Or you may decide that the benefits of the medication aren't worth the side effects and look for an alternative treatment.

Be sure you understand the directions on the labels. Some labels can be difficult to understand. For example, a lot of people don't know if taking a medication every four hours means you need to wake up and take it at night or if just taking it during the day is okay. If you're confused, ask the pharmacist for help. Pharmacists are a good resource for information on dosing, food and drug interactions, and which over-the-counter drugs might work best for you.

If the medicine is for a child, make sure you have the right dose and a good way to measure. Ask your pharmacist to double-check your child's weight with the dosage that was prescribed to make sure no mistakes were made. Remember that medication doses for children are calculated on body weight in *kilograms*, not pounds. Convert your child's weight yourself (divide his weight in pounds by 2.2 to find the weight in kilograms) and make sure the conversion and dosage were done correctly. Because of their small size and the immaturity of their organ systems, children are particularly susceptible to overdosing, so don't just assume, be *sure*.

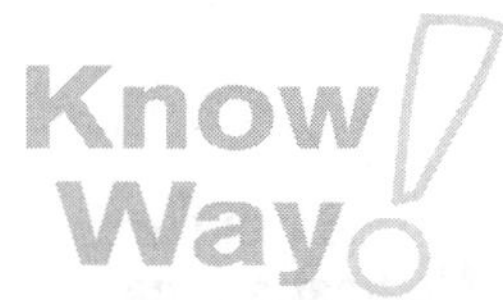

In one study, only 15 percent of emergency room patients over age sixty-five could correctly list all their medications and dosages.

Many reported medication errors occur in the hospital, so if you or someone you care about is in the hospital, be especially diligent about checking any medications that nurses or aides dispense. Even doctors themselves understand how severe this problem is. One surgeon whose wife was admitted to the hospital for several weeks reported that his wife experienced at least one attempted medication error every single day—sometimes more. A good rule of thumb is verify a medication with at least two different people (such as a nurse, a doctor, or an aide) and ask each of them twice to verify the medication and dosage and why you're taking it.

Make a list of all the prescription and over-the-counter medications you take and give a copy to your doctor, your pharmacist, and other health care professionals so they can keep your records up to date and give you better care. Take this list with you anytime you're going to the hospital or to any health facility for care.

What You Need to Know about the Drugs You Take

Know This	Example
Brand name of the drug	Tylenol, Warfarin, Floxin
Generic name of the drug	Acetaminophen, coumadin, ofloxacin
What type of drug is it?	Pain reliever, blood thinner, antibiotic
Dosage: how much and how often?	400 milligrams—one pill, two times a day
When do you take it?	10:00 A.M. and 6:00 P.M.
How do you take it?	Take on an empty stomach
Possible side effects	Dizziness, nausea, dry mouth
Possible interactions and precautions	Do not take with beta-blockers Do not drive after taking
Who prescribed it?	Doctor's name and phone number
Start and stop dates	June 6 to July 27, 2003
Any reactions you had	Experienced nausea and headaches Stopped taking because of side effects

How to use the Medication Log

Use this form to record the medication plan you have discussed with your doctor. List each drug you are supposed to take (including over-the-counter) and select a specific time for each dosage as shown in the sample below. Check off each dose you take. This will improve your chances of sticking to your schedule and getting the full benefits of the medication.

Drug Name *Acetaminophen*

Time	Dosage	Mon	Tue	Wed	Thu	Fri	Sat	Sun
2:00 pm	1 pill	✓	✓	✓	✓	✓	✓	✓
8:00 pm	2 pills	✓	✓		✓	✓		✓

Medication Log

Week beginning ______

Drug Name ______

Time	Dosage	Mon	Tue	Wed	Thu	Fri	Sat	Sun

Drug Name ______

Time	Dosage	Mon	Tue	Wed	Thu	Fri	Sat	Sun

Drug Name ______

Time	Dosage	Mon	Tue	Wed	Thu	Fri	Sat	Sun

Drug Name ______

Time	Dosage	Mon	Tue	Wed	Thu	Fri	Sat	Sun

vital sign 4 Your Health History

Take a few moments to ponder your life. Look back and reflect on your health. It's funny how many of the events in our life will trigger memories of our health and what we've experienced. Everyone remembers their first hospital stay. Images of doctors, orderlies, that 4:00 A.M. visit from the floor nurse. Think about how your health has changed over the course of your lifetime. When have you felt the best? What events put a strain on your health, either physical or mental? If you had any conditions that need ongoing treatment, have you followed up, or is there something that could use some attention?

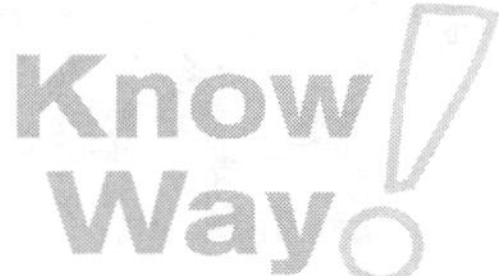

Mel Blanc, the man who was the voice of Bugs Bunny, was allergic to carrots.

Treatments you've undergone, procedures you've hated, illnesses you've beaten and those you still manage: as with most histories, often your past is the key to your future. Looking at your health history can help you see where your health challenges have come from and is

What You Need to Know about Your Health History

Know This	Example
What medical conditions do you have now or have had in the past?	Asthma, chest pains, migraines
Do you have any allergies?	Allergic to penicillin, strawberries, and bee stings
Did you have any childhood medical conditions?	Whooping cough, broken arm, hives
Medical tests and results	Sept. 2004, CBC (blood test)—normal March 1999, Pap smear—negative April 1998, Pap smear—negative March 1998, Pap smear—positive
Immunizations	Childhood, adult, and travel immunizations
Hospitalizations	Admission/discharge date, reason, physician, diagnosis, procedures, outcome, any complications and follow-up
Surgeries	Surgery date, procedure, hospital or facility, inpatient or outpatient, surgeon, tests, medications, complications
Illnesses and injuries	Date, ongoing or immediate, what caused it, physician, any complications, aftereffects, tests, medications, treatments

What You Need to Know about Your Critical Stats

Know This	When to Test
Weight	At least every three months
Blood pressure	If optimal, check every year If high, see chart on page 115
Cholesterol	If optimal, check every five years If high, check every year or more (ask your doctor)

often a good predictor of what may come in the future. A complete and honest health history will help your doctor determine what care you need now, which tests might be effective, and what has and hasn't worked for you in the past.

You'll also want to keep an ongoing history of your critical stats in the three areas shown to the left. Taking a measurement at the suggested frequency will let you and your doctor see trends in your health and also catch any problems before they get too far along.

If you are living with a health condition such as diabetes or asthma, you will also want to keep a history of your important stats in the areas that help you and your doctor manage your condition, for example, blood sugar levels and asthma peak flow records.

If there is something you are uncomfortable discussing with your doctor, having a written health history can make it a little easier to bring up. While it might make you nervous, being honest with your doctor is vital to allow her to make an accurate diagnosis and get you the right treatment. Also, tell your doctor that the topic makes you uncomfortable and why. Believe me, she has heard it all, and she can help you understand that the condition is not as uncommon as you think and is nothing to be embarrassed about. Knowing that you are uncomfortable will make her more understanding and, hopefully, more sensitive to your condition.

With the limited amount of time you get in most visits to your doctor, it's important that you bring up anything in your health history that might be significant without waiting for your doctor to ask. You don't have to cover every cold and sniffle, but major medical conditions will definitely be of interest to her in making a diagnosis, scheduling preventive screenings, and determining your future risks.

If you have an ongoing health condition that you manage, like diabetes, migraines, or arthritis, it's also a good idea to keep a written history of the treatments you have used and how they have worked. If you had a particular medication that just didn't do the trick, your

What You Need to Know about Blood Pressure Guidelines

Range	Reading	Checkup and Treatment
Optimal	less than 120/80	Check every year
Borderline	120/80–139/89	Check every six months Begin lifestyle changes
	High Blood Pressure Levels—See Your Doctor	
Mild	140/90–159/99	Check every two months Begin treatment
Moderate	160/100–179/109	Check every month Begin treatment within a month
Severe	over 180/110	Check every week Begin treatment within a week

What You Need to Know about Cholesterol Guidelines

	Optimal	Borderline	High Risk	Very High Risk
Total	under 200	200 to 239	240 and over	—
LDL (bad)	under 130	130 to 159	160 to 189	190 and over
HDL (good)	over 60	59 to 40	under 40	—
	Normal	**Borderline High**	**High**	**Very High**
Triglycerides	under 150	150 to 199	200 to 499	500+

doctor will need to know so that he doesn't try to prescribe it again. It also helps because some new medications are simply reformulations of older drugs. Your health history can be the key to unlocking many of the secrets of your health and will help you and your doctor forge a plan for a healthier future.

vital sign 5 Your Family Health History

If your health history holds the key to your future, the history of your family's health is the door you need to unlock. Scientists have known for a long time that your family history is one of the strongest predictors of your risk of developing any number of conditions, including asthma, diabetes, arthritis, Alzheimer's, allergies, and even vision or hearing loss, emotional conditions, and learning challenges. Now, with more and more genetic links to all types of conditions being discovered, the importance of your genetic makeup is becoming a critical part of staying healthy, finding conditions early, and discovering the keys to prevention.

What You Need to Know about Your Family's Health History

Record this information for as many family members as you can.

- Family member name
- Age or date of birth
- If no longer living, age at death
- If no longer living, cause of death
- Medical conditions
- Ethnic origin

Just as you can inherit your hair color, the color of your eyes, and even your personality traits, much of your health is passed down to you not just from your parents, but from generations of relations. Most of us, naturally, believe that our mother and father are the closest genetic links to our health. In fact, looking at the health of your brothers and sisters (born of the same mother and father) is much more telling, since they are the only other people in the world besides you with the unique combination of your mother's and father's genes.

Strange Things We Inherit

1. Color blindness
2. Baldness (from your mother!)
3. Ability to taste certain things
4. Ability to roll your tongue
5. Earlobes—attached or hanging

And it's not just heredity that falls from your family tree. Many of your healthstyle habits have come from the people you are closest to—usually your immediate family members. Where you live, what you eat, whether you smoke, your activity level—many of these traits can be traced back to habits you saw in your family members and developed yourself as a child. This can lead to a link in health conditions, not just through genetics but through the lifestyle choices you make as well.

The best way to gather information about your family health history is to talk about it to as many of your relatives as possible. Use the occasion of a family gathering to talk about your family's history or call your relatives to touch base. Explain what you are doing and promise to give each family a copy of the Family Health

History when you have completed it. Despite our candor about many parts of our lives, many people can be uncomfortable talking about their own health conditions or the conditions of family members. For some reason, we have developed a certain taboo in our culture against discussing health issues. While it's important to be aware of people's need for privacy about their health, at the same time, this taboo has kept us from openly discussing health issues that we should and made us uncomfortable about conditions, and often leads to a subtle feeling that a person is somehow to blame for a health condition.

Even your family's ethnic background can be important to diagnosing certain conditions. For example, people with a Mediterranean heritage may carry a gene for Mediterranean fever, a disease that runs in families and causes episodes of abdominal pain, arthritis, pleuritis, and peritonitis. If this heritage is unknown, often the pain is mistaken for appendicitis, resulting in an unnecessary appendectomy.

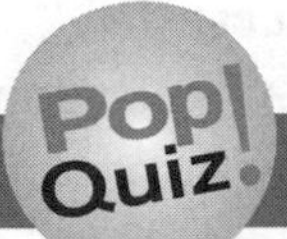

Your Vital Organs

1. This organ is six feet long and its major job is to remove salts and water from food.

   ____

2. Although essential to life, you can survive with less than one-half of this organ.

   ____

3. This controls activities that are not conscious, like balance and movement.

   ____

4. This organ expands and contracts fifteen times a minute.

   ____

5. This small organ produces insulin.

   ____

Answers

1. colon 2. liver 3. cerebellum 4. lung 5. pancreas

To paint the most complete portrait of your family, get information for as many relatives as you can, including the following.

Immediate family

- mother
- father
- sisters
- brothers

Extended family

- grandparents
- aunts, uncles, and first cousins
- nieces and nephews
- half-brothers and half-sisters

Ancestors

- great-grandparents
- great-aunts and great-uncles and more distant cousins

Some of the things to look for in your family history include:

- *Conditions that occur at an earlier age than normal*—before most people get the condition. Did Aunt Sarah get asthma at fifty-two or fourteen?

How to use the Family Health History

Use this form to record anyone in your family who has experienced a health condition. For those family members who are no longer living, record the cause of death under "Health Condition" if you know it. If you don't know much information about your family members, now is a good time to begin researching and recording this information for future generations.

Family Health History

Name ______________________________

Relationship	Name	Sex	Year Born/Died	Health Condition
			/	
			/	
			/	
			/	
			/	
			/	
			/	
			/	
			/	
			/	
			/	
			/	
			/	
			/	

- *Conditions in more than one close relative*—If you see heart disease in your father, brother, and an uncle, you will want to take extra steps to decrease your risks through diet and exercise and be sure to get preventive care and the tests you need.
- *Conditions that are unusual for a gender*—For example, if Uncle Ricardo died from breast cancer, you'll want to get screened for it earlier than usual.
- *Combinations of certain conditions within a family*—If both your mother and grandmother experienced both breast cancer and ovarian cancer, you may be carrying those genes. Talk to your doctor about gene counseling and how to asses your risk.

vital sign 6 Your Doctors

It's a good idea to keep contact records for every doctor you visit, even from the past. You never know when you will need to get old records or test results, and trying to recall who you saw several years ago, let alone their phone number or address, can be tough. This will also give you an understanding of your treatment and help you describe to your current doctor how your condition has been treated in the past. This information can also be invaluable if a condition reoccurs and you need to get your old records or talk to your former physician. Also include other health care professionals on your

RESOURCE

Is Your Doctor Certified?

See if your doctor has been board-certified at www.abms.org.

What You Need to Know about Your Doctors

Know This	Example
Name	Dr. Jason Schwartz
What is their specialty?	Cardiology
Address	Offices and clinics
Phone	Cell, office, fax, and e-mail
Office hours	9:00 A.M.–4:00 P.M. M–F, 9:00–11:00 A.M. Sat
What hospital do they use?	County General
Do they accept your insurance?	Accepts Well Cross, no Medicare
Special features	Four partners in office—can see someone else if my doctor is not available

list, such as your dentist, physical therapists, pharmacists, insurance brokers or contacts, hospitals, and anyone else you might need to contact about a health issue.

This information can also be critical in an emergency situation. Many hospitals are reluctant to give you care (other than that which will save your life) unless they can contact the doctor who's care you are under. This lets them make sure they aren't doing something that will undermine a treatment or endanger your life.

vital sign 7 Your Health Expenses

How can keeping track of your health expenses help you get better care? Well, unless you've got unlimited funds, which most of us don't, sooner or later, paying for your health can start to add up. By keeping tabs on how much you spend and what you spend it on, you can prioritize your health expenses and decide where your money would be used the best way.

What's an HSA?

Health Savings Accounts (HSAs) have been introduced as a new way to handle your rising health care expenses. Here are some facts to help you figure them out.

1. **What is an HSA?** A Health Savings Account (HSA) is a bank account that you put money into to help you pay for health care expenses that are not covered by your insurance.
2. **What is the benefit of putting money into an HSA?** You do not pay taxes on the money in the account. The money you don't use can stay in the account and roll over tax-free (as the law stands now).
3. **Can anyone have an HSA?** No. To qualify you have to have what's called a "high-deductible" health plan, where you are responsible for paying for a portion of your medical expenses before your insurance plan will pay. The deductible amount does not include your monthly premium.
4. **What qualifies as a high-deductible plan?** A plan where your deductible amount (what you have to pay for office visits, hospital stays, or medications) is at least $1,050 and no more than $5,250 for an individual and at least $2,100 and no more than $10,500 for a family. So you have to be prepared to pay at least $2,100 (or more) for your family's medical expenses before any insurance benefits will kick in.
5. **Is there a limit on how much you can put into the HSA?** Yes. Right now you are limited to $2,700 per year for an individual and $5,450 for a family. Of course, you can save more, but it won't be tax-free.

I advise you to talk with your employer health benefits rep, financial advisor, or insurance agent to see if an HSA is right for you.

What You Need to Know about Your Health Expenses

Know This	Example
Life insurance	Company, policy number, coverage, benefit amount, premiums, phone number
Health insurance	Company, policy number, coverage, benefits, premiums, phone number, primary care physicians and number of members covered, main subscriber
Other insurance	Vision insurance, dental insurance, or other supplemental insurance
Medical expenses	Date of service, what was done, who provided the service, amount, how you paid, deductible

In addition to the responsibility for making decisions about your health, more and more of the responsibility for paying for your health care is being shifted to you, whether you have a health insurance plan or not. Deductibles keep rising, while maximum payouts seem to be getting lower and lower. New Health Savings Accounts (HSAs) offer you a way to pay for your health expenses with money placed into a special account. These HSAs are used along with high-deductible insurance plans that lower the monthly premiums you have to pay by a lot, but also make you responsible for all your health care expenses until they reach a high amount like $5,000 per year, called your deductible. If you are relatively healthy and don't use many health services, this can amount to a big cost savings. But the trade-off is that you pay for everything until your expenses go over that deductible amount.

New choices like these are giving consumers more power to make their own decisions about how their health care dollar is spent, but also mean that you've got to become a lot more aware of what services for your health can cost and make educated choices about how you're going to spend that money. And you may be in for some sticker shock when the bills start rolling in. I heard one such story from Bill, who owns a small donut shop with his wife, Alycia, in New Mexico.

> Our health insurance premiums had just gotten, to put it bluntly, unaffordable. We've got three small children and since we're self-employed, we pay for our own health insurance. We

were already struggling to pay the $950 monthly premium when we got a letter from the insurance company saying our premium would be going up to $1,175! Alycia nearly fainted. She keeps the books and she said we just couldn't afford to pay that much anymore. We were frustrated because our kids are five, nine, and eleven and are pretty darn healthy. Aside from yearly checkup exams for school and an occasional flu or rash, we hardly ever went to the doctor at all. We really just wanted insurance in case Alycia or me got sick or one of the kids had an accident or needed an operation for something serious. I called our insurance broker and asked him to see if there was anything he could do.

He showed me some new options that had just come up—plans with a really high deductible but low monthly premiums. He said that I could set up a Health Savings Account, put pretax money into it, and pay for any health expenses out of there. The good thing is that the money would roll over from year to year and if we didn't use it we could put it toward retirement

5 minute clinic

6 Ways to Find Cheap Prescription Drugs

1. **Shop around.** Drug prices can vary more than 200 percent from store to store, so shop around for each of your drugs. Also, many drugstores, retailers, and club stores like Wal-Mart, Target, and Costco are responding to consumer demand for cheaper drugs with major discount programs.
2. **Check out state and community programs.** Some states offer programs to make medicines affordable to those who demonstrate a need. Check with community health centers, Area Agencies on Aging, or your state health agency.
3. **Visit www.needymeds.com.** If you're looking for help with your prescriptions, look here first. You can look up individual drugs and drug company patient assistant programs and even print out applications for various Patient Assistance Programs (called PAPs).
4. **Consider generic drugs.** As long as your doctor approves, using a generic drug rather than a brand name will cut your cost considerably, and by law, generics must be just as effective. But be aware that not every drug has a generic equivalent.
5. **Call the drug manufacturer.** Almost every pharmaceutical company has a Patient Assistance Program. The list of companies is too long to include here, but ask your doctor or go to www.needymeds.com on the Internet and click on Company List on the left.
6. **Ask your doctor for help.** Some Patient Assistance Programs require that your doctor file an application for you. Your doctor may also know of programs that will help you get the drugs you need at a cost you can afford.

or pay for health insurance after we retired. The best part was our premiums would go down to $210 a month!

I was a little worried about the $10,000 deductible amount, but Alycia said, "We have some savings and you know, we could take out a loan on the shop if something drastic happens. As long as the insurance would kick in after $10,000, I think we could handle that. And after a couple of years of putting money into the Health Savings Account, we should be able to build it up to use in case something serious comes up. Besides, we'll be saving almost $12,000 in premiums a year. For that amount we can pay for our health care when we need it."

Well, that convinced me and I signed us up. Everything was fine. Our new policy even gave us discount rates for prescription drugs and free checkups once a year. And it took a lot of pressure off us financially not to have to pay those high premiums every month.

Several months into the plan, Alycia noticed that she was feeling particularly tired. She had always been anemic, but it seemed to be worse than usual. She went to the doctor for a checkup. The doctor wasn't worried, but wanted to run a few tests just to make sure everything was okay. Alycia paid the doctor's $75 office visit charge—no sweat! That was certainly worth what we were saving in premiums every month. Alycia's test came back A-OK and the doctor told her to try some iron pills for a couple of months. A few weeks later a bill arrived from the lab where Alycia's doctor had sent her tests. $750! Sticker shock!

Did I read that right? $750 for a little test? I mean, when I take my car in for work, my mechanic looks it over and then calls me and says, "It's going to be $275 to fix your starter." I think I even have to sign some kind of approval to do the work. I asked Alycia if the doctor had told her the test would be that much. "No," she said, "he didn't say anything about it or ask me if I wanted it or anything."

We weren't mad at the doctor, we just had no idea how expensive these things were—our insurance company had always just paid. I mean, considering what we were saving on our insurance premiums, it was still a great deal and I am glad

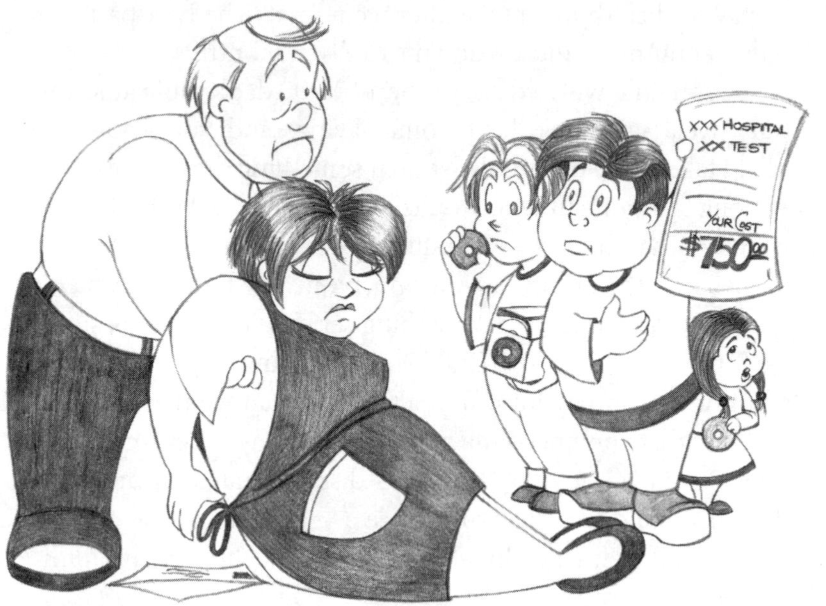

we found out that Alycia was okay. It's sure better to pay $750 for a test now than to let some condition develop and have it be serious and cost even more down the line. We just learned that we better ask before just letting things be done and be prepared to pay more than we'd expect. Alycia even mentioned it to her doctor at her next appointment and he said, "I never thought about it, but you're right. Now that patients are paying for things themselves, I really ought to let them know and make sure they understand what it will cost beforehand. This is a whole new way of dealing with care."

Experts say that one of the biggest problem controlling costs in our health care system is that nobody knows what anything costs. This keeps you not only from shopping around or making informed decisions on how to spend your health care dollar, but makes competition based on price and quality virtually nonexistent. Understanding where your health care dollar goes will help make the system more efficient and let you decide what your health priorities are and how your health dollars are spent.

As you pay for more of your own health care, the most important thing you can do for both your health and your wallet is to be sure

Evaluating Your Health Plan

Use this chart to gather information about your current health plan or evaluate a new plan. If your agent or employer representative doesn't know the answers, try calling the plan's customer service line.

If prescription drugs are a significant part of your health care expenses, you'll want to get exact details on how a plan covers those copayments. Some plans have very complex structures for drugs based on brand names, generics, mail order, and so on. The best thing is to make a list of the drugs you take regularly and ask the agent or health plan representative to tell you exactly how much you can expect to pay a month.

Seeing Doctors

Plan Name ______________________________

Where can I choose my doctor from? ☐ Plan list of doctors ☐ Any doctor

Do I have to pay extra to use a doctor outside the plan? ☐ YES ☐ NO

How much? ______________________________

How often can I change doctors? ______________________________

Can I use my current doctor for an ongoing condition? ☐ YES ☐ NO

What is the limit on the number of office visits in a year? ______________________________

Does the plan pay for a second opinion? ☐ YES ☐ NO

Do I need a referral from my doctor to see a specialist? ☐ YES ☐ NO

Plan Services

What is the limit for hospital stays? ______________________________

Is my preexisting condition covered? ☐ YES ☐ NO

Does the plan cover preventive services? ☐ YES ☐ NO

Do I have to get approval for emergency treatment? ☐ YES ☐ NO

Can I order drugs online or through mail order? ☐ YES ☐ NO

Am I covered when I travel out of state? ☐ YES ☐ NO

Costs

What's the plan deductible? ______________________________

What's my maximum out-of-pocket expense? ______________________________

Does it qualify for an HSA? ______________________________

What's the copayment for an office visit? ______________________________

What's the copayment for a hospital stay? ______________________________

What's the maximum the plan will cover in a year? ______________________________

Pop Quiz! Money, Money, Money

Take a guess at what you think each of these services or procedures cost:

1. Emergency Room visit $__________
2. Doctor's office visit $__________
3. Mammogram $__________
4. Appendectomy $__________
5. Heart transplant $__________

Answers

1. $390 2. $60 3. $100 4. $5,000 5. $250,000

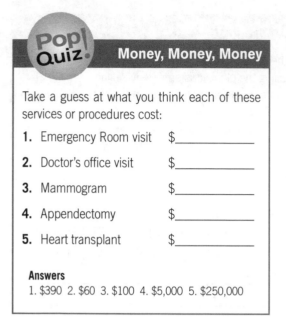

and put some funds aside in your budget for preventive care—checkups, screenings, fitness, even nutritional counseling if you want to lose some weight. Believe me, investing in good health early will pay off big, not only in minimizing surprise medical expenses, but more importantly, in catching conditions as early as possible to make treatment easier and save your life.

Surveys of Americans say that the cost of health care is the leading topic of concern. Over half the personal bankruptcies filed in this country are a result of overwhelming medical expenses. Over 45 million people (and counting) aren't covered by health insurance, a large portion of those being children. Even those who have insurance are watching benefits shrink and copayments and deductibles go up. There's lots of options for coverage out there, so whether you have coverage through your employer or buy it on your own, take the time to evaluate your plan and know the benefits. It also helps to understand what's covered and what you'll be responsible for paying yourself. This will let you use all of the benefits your plan covers, like free checkups or health education classes to stay as healthy as possible.

Taylor's Fifth Law of Health

Having a health plan is not the same as planning for your health.

Prescription 4

Plan for Your life

Your Money or Your Life

Charlie Bell had a great plan for his career. At fifteen, on a bus ride home from school in his native Australia, he ran into a friend going to apply for a job at the local McDonald's. Charlie's friend wasn't hired, but Charlie was. Bell dropped out of school at age fifteen to take that job behind the counter, and by nineteen he was the youngest McDonald's store manager in Australia. By thirty-one he was appointed the managing director of McDonald's Australia operation and had a beautiful wife and new baby daughter, Alex. Finally, at age forty-four, Charlie had fulfilled his lifelong dream, rising to the position of President and CEO of the McDonald's Corporation. Two weeks after his appointment to his new position, Bell was diagnosed with colorectal cancer. Nine months later Charlie Bell was dead.

Since it is slow-growing, the survival rate for colorectal cancer can be greater than 90 percent if caught early. The devastating tragedy is that Charlie Bell might still be alive today if he had planned for his health the way he planned for his career.

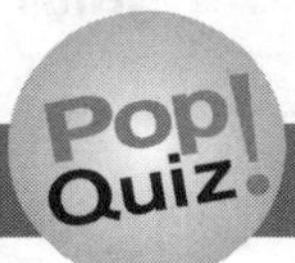

Aches and Pains

1. Joint pain is the leading cause of disability in people under forty-five. True False
2. You should put ice on a strained ankle. True False
3. Most back pain is caused by a spinal abnormality. True False
4. Tension headaches are the most common type of headache. True False
5. Arthritis can cause hoarseness. True False

Answers

1. False. Back pain is.
2. True. The rule of thumb is "Ice a strain (acute), heat a pain (chronic)."
3. False. Most back pain is caused by a muscle strain and will get better in a few weeks.
4. True. They account for three-quarters of all headaches.
5. True. Arthritis can affect the joints in the vocal cords, but it is usually not dangerous.

In Bell's final months, McDonald's Corporation spent more than $300,000 to fly Bell and his family back to Australia on a private jet specially equipped to provide him with medical care and bought his home in Illinois for over $600,000. The average cost for the test to detect colon cancer (a colonoscopy) is about $600.

Think about what's more important to you, your money or your health? I believe most of us would put more value on our health than on most of our possessions. It doesn't take much of an illness or physical setback for someone to realize how much it's worth to have good health and feel well. Yet ask any American if they've got a health plan, and those who are insured will answer, "Yeah, I'm with Blue Cross (or Wellpoint or HealthNet)." If you say, "No, a plan for how you're going to stay healthy," you'll get "Huh?" It's great to have health insurance, but that's planning for your financial well-being, not your health.

Ironically, your money and your health are tied more closely than you might guess. In its February 2006 issue, *Smart Money* magazine laid out how to accumulate one million dollars. At the top of their list? Taking care of your health. The article's author goes on to say that health expenses, especially unexpected ones, are one of the biggest threats to your financial well-being.

Control your destiny or somebody else will.

—JACK WELCH, FORMER CEO OF GENERAL ELECTRIC

Experts say that making a few small changes in the way we mange our health could save countless lives every year. In his popular financial planning book, *Think and Grow Rich*, author Napoleon Hill wrote that 85 percent of all failures result from not having a sense of purpose. But in our society planning for your health is virtually unheard of, resulting in needless deaths and devastated families like Charlie Bell's. It's not that we're lazy and won't do what it takes to protect our health. I believe it's because we've never had a road map for how to manage our health. We grow up being told we need to be responsible with our money, with our house, with our jobs, with our children, but no one ever tells you how to be responsible with our health. So what's out there to help you?

Do-It-Yourself Health

Diet and exercise, by far, dominate the health resources I uncovered, from books to Internet sites to video and even podcasts. If the number of diet and exercise books were any indication, you'd think we'd be a much healthier nation! If you're having trouble losing weight and getting in shape, it's certainly not for a lack of information, although I wonder—could it in fact be because there's just too much info (and food) to digest?

But go to the Internet bookstore Amazon.com and search for "Financial Planning." You'll get over 4,500 results. Most people understand that when it comes to your money, some type of planning helps—balance your checkbook, pay your bills on time, save for retirement. But even people who manage their bank accounts penny by penny probably don't have any kind of plan when it comes to their health.

Now go to Amazon and search for "Health Planning." There are lots of books aimed at government and public agencies on how to plan public health programs. But, in fact, I didn't find any books that individuals could use to help develop a plan to protect or improve the state of their health.

If you bought a house and didn't lift one finger to do maintenance or check the systems on that house for ten years, you wouldn't expect the house to be in tip-top shape, would you? If all of a sudden it started springing leaks in the roof and had termites and the air conditioning system stopped working, you would think, "Well, I guess I should have taken better care of it." It's just common sense.

Your body is the same way. Our bodies are actually quite amazing things. We get sick—we get better. We cut our skin—it heals. We throw out our back—we rest, and the pain subsides. We get the flu—our immune system attacks it. But when you start to take this amazing machine

RESOURCE

Healthy Living Calculators

Measure everything from BMI to calories to ovulation at www.brighamandwomens.org/healthinfo/healthtools.asp.

4 Health Products That Really Work

1. Motion sickness wristbands
2. Vicks VapoRub for chest congestion
3. Nicotine aids. Ask your doctor about side effects, but these have helped many people quit smoking.
4. Hydrocortisone cream to heal small skin irritations, sores, and blemishes (use sparingly)

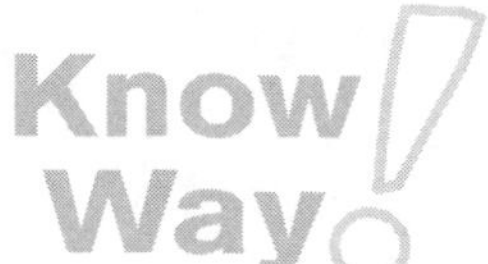

Health officials report that two-thirds of Americans don't get an annual physical checkup.

for granted, when you expect that you don't have to do any maintenance, don't have to get any checkups, don't have to monitor your systems, how can you be surprised when you start springing leaks, so to speak?

And just like with a house, once that water starts pouring through your roof, you either do major repairs, get a new roof, or pray for no rain. Now if you had taken care of that roof—patched small holes, replaced shingles—along the way, you probably wouldn't need a new one. But now, well . . . it just can't be saved. Again, just like your body. If you do some maintenance, get some tests, get preventive care, you can patch the holes while they're still small. Slightly elevated blood pressure at thirty? Try changing your diet and getting some exercise. Dangerously high blood pressure at sixty-five? Now you're talkin' major medications and a high risk of a heart attack. Got a small lump? Let's take it out and biopsy. Stage 1 cancer: Remove the tumor, maybe radiation; full recovery likely. But undetected tumor for four years? Radiation to shrink it; try to remove it, probably major chemotherapy.

I'm not saying it's all under your control. Just like earthquakes, hurricanes, and tornadoes, the unexpected sometimes happens. But your first line of defense is a good offense. And even in a natural disaster, people with an emergency plan are prepared and know what to do. It's no different for your health. You just need a great plan so you know what to do and when to do it. You don't have to give up your life to be healthy. I just don't want you to give up your health for your life.

Pop Quiz! **Diabetes**

1. Craving sweets is a symptom of diabetes. True False
2. Type 2 diabetes will eventually turn into type 1 diabetes. True False
3. Type 2 diabetes is an inherited condition. True False
4. All people with diabetes must take insulin. True False
5. Pregnancy is dangerous if you have diabetes. True False

Answers

1. False. Eating sugar has nothing to do with diabetes.
2. False. Type 1 and type 2 diabetes are two entirely different conditions caused by different things. The type of diabetes you have does not change because of weight gain or loss, diet, or age.
3. False. Being overweight is the primary cause of type 2 diabetes.
4. False. Everyone with type 1 diabetes must take insulin. People who have type 2 diabetes only take insulin if their condition cannot be controlled through diet and exercise.
5. False. Pregnancy is no more dangerous for women with diabetes as long as they manage their blood sugar and get early treatment for any complications.

Is There Going to Be a Quiz on This?

Was Charlie Bell negligent in not planning for his health? Was he too focused on his career to worry about getting preventive screenings and checkups? I didn't know Charlie Bell, but if he was like the rest of us, the answer is "*no*." Once someone has been diagnosed with a condition, it's easy to say, "If only he'd gotten this test" or "If she'd only had a checkup, it might have been caught sooner." Anyone who's ever gotten bad news at the doctor's office, without a doubt, will wonder on the drive home, "Could I have done something to find this sooner?" But we can't blame ourselves. The fact is, our health system does little, if anything, to help us understand how to manage or have a plan for our health.

For decades doctors have been in charge of our care—primarily because they wanted it that way. We jumped right from having a family doctor who made house calls and knew all the children by name to having a different primary care physician every six months assigned to you by your HMO. I think most of us were absent the day they handed out the textbook *How to Manage Your Own Health*. There are so many options for care today that when you're diagnosed with a health condition, you're not only faced with the diagnosis, but have to become an instant expert on your health—making decisions about treatment, deciding if you need a second opinion, researching options

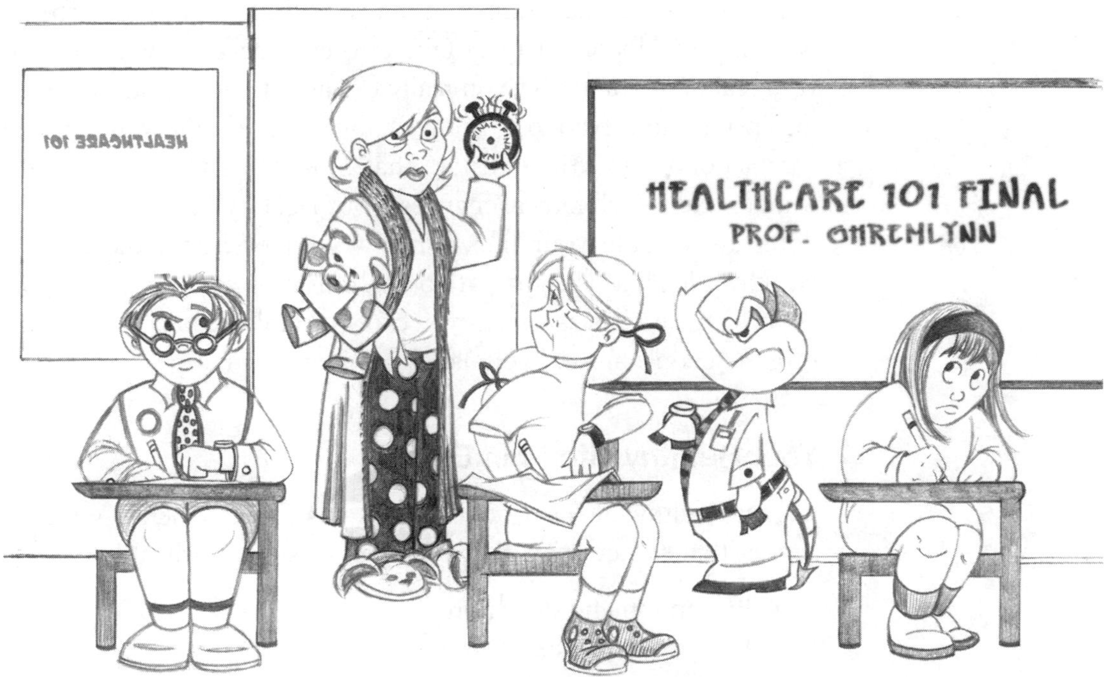

for care, and on and on. It's as if that popular nightmare about school has come true—you show up for class only to find that it's the last day of class, you've slept through the whole year, and now you've got to take your final exam—except this exam is life and death.

We've learned to accept this lack of planning and care as just par for the course. I asked a doctor once if he'd ever gotten a postcard from his auto mechanic saying, "It's time for your car's yearly oil change"?

"Of course," he replied, "I get them all the time."

"So," I asked, "why don't doctors send out reminders to their patients that it's time for a checkup, or time to get that mammogram, or Billy's immunization is due? Don't you think that's just a little more important than making sure your car's running right?"

"I guess we just don't think of health that way," was his answer.

But if our doctors aren't thinking that way, who is? Looks like it's up to you.

Your Healthy Life Plan

Developing your Healthy Life Plan isn't hard. The plan isn't a phone-book-size research paper filled with technical medical details. The key is to make it doable. It must take into consideration your real life, your real habits, and how you really feel about your health. Developing an ambitious plan to radically change your life and your health is commendable, but the odds are that most of us just can't or don't want to make such radical changes. Your Healthy Life Plan shouldn't dominate or rule your life; rather, your life should dictate your Healthy Life Plan. The goal is to be as healthy as you can, feel as good as you can, and live as long as you can so that you can enjoy your life, love the people around you, laugh a lot, and be happy.

Your Healthy Life Plan Basics

In your Healthy Life Plan, you'll write a mission statement—goals and actions that should include two major areas of your health:

- Prevention and detection
- Healthstyle habits

Prevention and Detection

The key to prevention is to identify your health risks and take the steps to keep you from getting health conditions or detect those you can't prevent as early as possible so that treatment is simple and effective. The Personal Health Assessment that you completed in the previous chapter is a great tool to help you identify your areas of risk and address them in your Healthy Life Plan. But don't just count on the risks that show up in your Personal Health Assessment. Not every condition has a link to heredity, lifestyle choices, or the like, so it's critical for your Healthy Life Plan to include basic screenings.

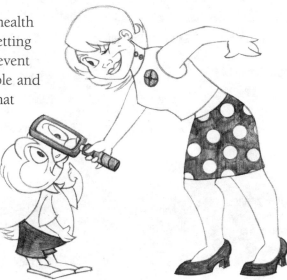

Everyone should have a schedule of the preventive screenings and exams that are currently recommended. The Checklist of Preventive Screenings on page 134 lists screenings that are recommended by the U.S. Preventive Services Task Force for healthy adults. You can use these handy charts to list the date for your next screening or exam then check it off once you've completed it. The checklist will help you when you develop your Healthy Life Plan by telling you what you should have done and when. While some of these screenings are momentarily unpleasant, trust me, it's a blip on the radar compared to the upside of finding out that you're free and clear. That's the funny thing about our avoidance of tests. Not having a test doesn't make a condition go away, it just makes the treatment more of a challenge once it's finally discovered. Don't go into a screening afraid of what you'll find. Go in happy knowing that the test is merely going to confirm your good health. It's just as easy to see that glass as half full and will reduce your anxiety at the same time.

RESOURCE

Printable Guide of Adult Screenings

Geared to the medical professional, but still useful: visit www.ahrq.gov/clinic/pocketgd.htm.

Remember that the checklist of preventive screenings is just the basics. You'll also want to review your Health History and Family Health History with your doctor and talk about anything else that could reveal other health risks. There may be additional screenings or exams that you and your doctor may decide are right for you based on your specific health factors. For example, if you have a family

Checklist of Preventive Screenings and Exams			
My Date	**Exam or Screening**	**Should Include**	**When**
	Physical Exam	Skin exam, blood pressure, cholesterol, urinalysis, and blood sugar	Every one to three years
	Dental Exam	Talk to your dentist about conditions that could affect your teeth or gums, like diabetes	Every year
	Vision Test	Glaucoma every four years, every two years after age sixty-five or if you have a family history	Every one to three years
	Hearing Test	Test for hearing impairment	Every one to three years
	Blood Pressure	Keep a log of results	Every year
	Cholesterol	Keep a log of results	Every five years
	Fecal Blood Occult	Screens for colorectal cancer	Every year after age fifty
	Sigmoidoscopy	Screens for colorectal cancer and bowel conditions	Every five years after age fifty
	Colonoscopy	Used when early screenings indicate a risk	Every ten years after age fifty

history of early heart disease or you have several risk factors, you may want to get a stress test to determine if there is adequate blood flow to your heart or if you have any blockages.

Healthstyle Habits

Good healthstyle habits means living life to the fullest while making good choices. Think about what you want to do to minimize the negative effects any health conditions have on your ability to live your

Screenings for Men		
My Date	**Exam or Screening**	**When**
	Digital Rectal Exam	Every year after age thirty-nine
	Prostate Exam	Every year
	PSA Blood Test	Every year after age fifty, sooner if risk suspected
	Testicular Exam	Every year by physician, self-exam monthly
	Heart Disease	Discuss prevention at checkup
	Impotence	Discuss if issue
	Depression	Discuss if issue
	Infertility	Discuss if issue

Screenings for Women		
My Date	**Exam or Screening**	**When**
	PAP Smear	Every three years if normal result
	Pelvic Exam	Every year
	Mammogram	Every two years after age forty, every year after age fifty
	Breast Exam	Every year by physician, self-exam monthly
	Bone Density Test	Every five years after age sixty-five; earlier if risk factors
	Heart Disease	Discuss prevention at checkup
	Birth Control	Discuss if issue
	Infertility	Discuss if issue
	Depression	Discuss if issue
	Menopause	Discuss at age forty-five or if you experience symptoms

Keep in mind that you may need other tests and screenings that are not listed here based on your health conditions, health history, and family history.

These lists are just a starting point for your healthy life. If you get a test result that shows an abnormal result—high blood pressure, high cholesterol, elevated PSA level—don't just leave it there. Work with your doctor to develop a treatment plan and also see what other tests you might need to figure out how your health is being affected and what you can do to cure and treat your condition.

Other Common Tests and Screenings		
Exam or Screening	**What It Is**	**When**
EKG (Electrocardiogram)	Small sensors are used to diagnose abnormalities in your heart functions	If you are at risk for heart disease or have unexplained chest pains
Angiogram	X-rays of coronary arteries used to detect blockages and assess function of heart valves	If your doctor suspects blockages or you have severe chest pains
Complete Blood Count (CBC)	Blood test to measure the number and size of different types of blood cells	To assess general health and detect certain conditions
Chest X-ray	X-ray of chest area	If you are at risk for lung cancer, smoke, or have difficulty breathing
Skin Biopsy	A small sample of skin is removed and tested for cancer	If a mole or other skin marking has changed color or size or is cause for concern
Blood Sugar	Tests for elevated blood glucose levels in your blood	Every three years or if you are at risk for diabetes
HIV (Human Immunodeficiency Virus) Test	Test to determine if an HIV infection is present in your blood	The CDC has issued a recommendation that an HIV test become a standard screening for everyone ages thirteen to sixty-four
Thyroid Hormone	Blood test to check for thyroid function or hypothyroidism (up to 10 percent of women may experience hypothyroidism)	If you have symptoms such as unexplained weight gain, dry skin, fatigue, cold skin, or other risks

life. Consider where you can make positive choices that will help you feel good about yourself and your health and keep you safe and protected.

You can't have the perfect Healthy Life Plan in a split second. Everyone knows what happens to New Year's resolutions starting on January 2! That's because we try to take on too much, too soon. You don't have to change everything all at once. Choose a couple of areas where you'd like to make improvements and set some goals for those. Doctors can be intimidating when it comes to setting your health goals, which is why it's important for you to think about them on your own, then get your doctor's input. Doctors often want to fix everything at once, trying to get you to some perfect state of health. This can be overwhelming for a lot of us, hearing that you're overweight, your blood pressure is up, your cholesterol is high, and oh, by the way, you're anemic, too!

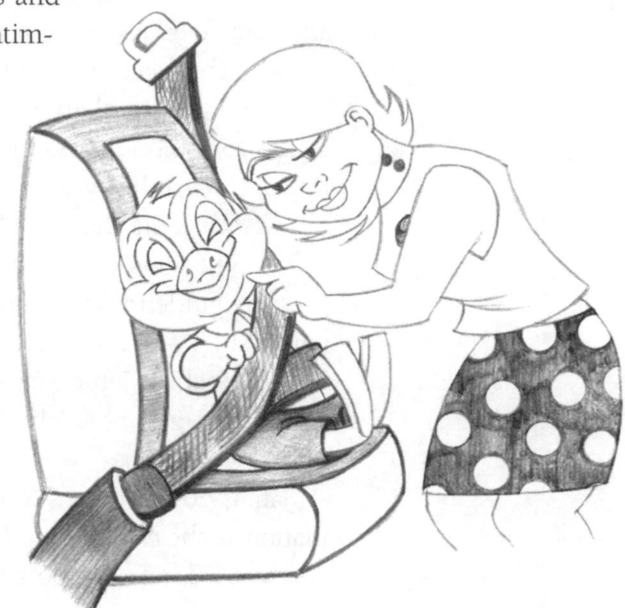

How Can I Win If You Keep Changing the Rules of the Game?

After having two children and struggling with her weight for years, Janie decided that this was the year she was going to get healthy. She found a plan that helped her count her calories and within three months had lost thirty pounds! Although she hadn't given up soda or an occasional hot fudge sundae, she had changed the way she was eating, choosing smaller portions, getting more fruits and vegetables, and sticking (most days) to her daily calorie allowance. She felt good about herself, had more energy, and finally fit into those size-8 jeans!

When the time came nine months later for her yearly physical, for the first time she could remember, she was actually looking forward to it.

"Great," Dr. Simmons said, "you've lost some weight. How'd you do it?"

"I gave myself a daily calorie limit and then just stuck with it," Janie said, beaming.

"No exercise?"

A little deflated, Janie said, "No, not really. I mean, with two kids in school and a full-time job, there's not much time to go to the gym."

Nodding, Dr. Simmons said, "I know it's tough, but the new guidelines from the government recommend ninety minutes of exercise a

The Most Dangerous Appliances in Your Home

- Space heaters: fire hazard, burns, carbon monoxide
- Stoves: burns, fires
- Clothes dryers: fire hazard from lint trap
- Electric mixers: finger injuries, projectile hazard (spoons, knives)
- Irons: burns, fires

day. You know, you might start to gain that weight back if you don't add some exercise to your routine."

Janie shrugged, noticeably disappointed, and said, "Okay."

Looking at the chart in her lap, Dr. Simmons said, "The good news is that your blood pressure's come down from the mild hypertensive range it was at last year."

"Great," Janie thought, "at least I'm doing something right!"

Dr. Simmons continued, "The bad news is that the new blood pressure guidelines now put you in the 'Prehypertensive' category, so you're still in a danger zone."

"Oh, really?" Janie thought. "Funny, I can feel my blood pressure going up right now," but thought better of actually voicing this opinion.

Janie's doctor means well. She's trying to give Janie as much information as she can, to help Janie make good health care decisions. But is that working? A report in *USA Today* quotes Dr. Steven Woolf, a

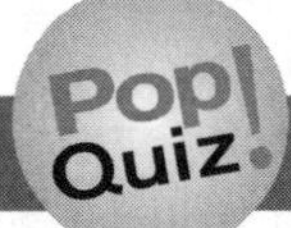

Count Your Calories

Circle the food with the most calories on each line:

1. 3 oz. hamburger 3 oz. chicken 4 oz. tuna hot dog

2. bagel slice of bread hot dog bun bowl of corn flakes

3. corn avocado potato cauliflower

4. chocolate bar cupcake fudge pop 1 tsp. sugar

5. light beer black coffee tea soda

6. cheddar cheese 2% milk yogurt whole egg

Answers

Note: All calories are approximate based on a single-serving size. Brands and preparation methods can affect calories.

1. hamburger, 220 hot dog, 190 tuna, 180 chicken, 120
2. bagel, 150 hot dog bun, 140 corn flakes, 110 bread, 80
3. avocado, 300 corn (1 ear), 100 potato, 100 cauliflower, 15
4. chocolate bar, 270 cupcake, 165 fudge pop, 60 sugar, 15
5. soda, 140 beer, 90 black coffee, 4 tea, 2
6. yogurt, 240 2% milk, 120 cheddar cheese, 110 egg, 75

primary care physician and a member of the U.S. Preventive Services Task Force: "It's already a difficult enough challenge for patients to lose a few pounds, to adopt a regular exercise program. Calling it prehypertension doesn't make it any easier."

That's why developing your Healthy Life Plan is so important. You develop the goals that mean something to you and are based on your risk factors, health history, family history, and, most importantly, what you want out of your health and your life. You can use the guidelines issued by the U.S. government, talk to your doctor about what they recommend, and do as much research as you like on prevention, illness, or alternative therapies. But the important thing is that your goals reflect what you want, not arbitrary changes in standards or sensational Headline Health. This gives you the strength and the power to help your doctor understand what's important to you, what you're willing and not willing to do, and your commitment to protecting your life and your health.

Developing Your Healthy Life Plan Goals and Actions

Think about your goals and the actions you will take to achieve those goals. Look at the "whys," not just the "hows," of staying healthy. It's easy to dash off a few standard goals—lose twenty pounds, get more exercise, eat better. But take a few minutes to look back at your Life Priorities Audit. Review your Health Fears Appraisal. Until you figure out why you want to be healthy and what commitment you're willing to make, you can't come up with realistic goals that fit your life—not some diet guru's or magazine editor's. Your reasons can be simple—to live longer, to be able to travel, to look good, to be alive for my children. Keeping it simple will help you make these goals an everyday part of your life.

Setting goals will help propel you into action and also give you a clear sign of when you've reached your goals. Focusing on specific actions you can take will also make more of an impact on how you feel and your overall health. Lots of people make a vow on January 1 of every year ("This is the year I take better care of my heart") but don't have a clear picture of what that means or exactly how they plan to accomplish it. If you've pinpointed a certain area of your health

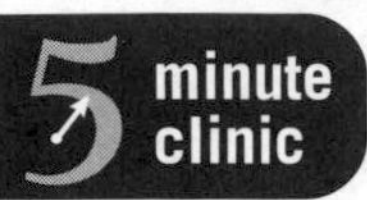

8 Questions to Ask Yourself about a Goal

1. **Do I have the information I need to achieve the goal?** If you answer "yes," make sure that the information is available to you or you understand where you can find it.
2. **What help do I need to make this goal happen?** Write down assistance or support you need to achieve your goal and the people or organizations who may be able to help.
3. **Are there any resources or skills that I need?** Do you need any training, outside resources, or skills to achieve your goal? Make getting those skills and resources one of your first action steps.
4. **Is the goal a challenge?** Setting a goal that's too easily achieved is a waste of your time.
5. **Does achieving this goal depend on someone else?** It's okay to get help from others, but if your goal depends on someone else, you may be setting yourself up for failure if that person doesn't come through.
6. **What will keep me from achieving this goal?** By exploring the possible roadblocks, you can start working on strategies for overcoming the difficulties without getting discouraged.
7. **Is this goal achievable or am I taking on too much?** Even goals that seem unachievable to others can be reached with the right determination, planning, and devotion. Be realistic about what you take on, considering all of the responsibilities in your life. Make sure you don't have too many lofty goals or you are apt to abandon them all.
8. **What if I reach my goal?** Asking this question can help you be sure you're striving toward something you really want.

that you'd like to work on (managing your diabetes, losing weight, getting treatment for your migraine headaches), knowing and listing the exact steps you can take to manage that condition or just be healthier will give you a plan you can follow—not just vague hopes and wishes. Your Healthy Life Plan will give you an easy-to-follow set of action steps so you know where you're going, which path to follow, what to do to get there, and how you'll know when you've arrived.

Most of us just take our health for granted. But think about your health milestones the same way you approach other milestones in your life—college, marriage, buying a house, having kids. Do the same for your health. Plan, prepare for, and execute your health goals to help you reach your ultimate goal—a lifetime of good health.

Healthy Life Plan—Milestone 20s

A major focus should be to establish healthy eating and exercise habits and begin good preventive health measures. If you have weight issues, now is the time to address them—it will get harder as you get older. If you have any health conditions, it's also the best time to learn as much as you can about them and start good management routines.

HEALTH PLAN FOR YOUR

20s

Mission Statement: ____________________

____

Sample: Maintain a healthy weight, establish an exercise routine, and identify and minimize unhealthy habits.

Goal ____________________

Actions

- ____________
- ____________
- ____________
- ____________
- ____________
- ____________

Goal ____________________

Actions

- ____________
- ____________
- ____________
- ____________
- ____________
- ____________

Goal ____________________

Actions

- ____________
- ____________
- ____________
- ____________
- ____________
- ____________

Goal ____________________

Actions

- ____________
- ____________
- ____________
- ____________
- ____________
- ____________

Goal ____________________

Actions

- ____________
- ____________
- ____________
- ____________
- ____________
- ____________

Example:

Goal *Limit alcohol*

Actions *no mixed drinks*

2 drinks per day max

no prepartying

1 month dry each year

Prevention and Detection

- Checkup (every three years)
- Dental exam (every year)
- Tetanus booster
- HPV vaccination (women)
- Rubella (women)

Just for men: Testicular cancer is the most common malignancy in men ages fifteen to thirty-four. Do a self-exam every month.

Healthstyle Habits to Consider

- Smoking or tobacco use
- Recreational drug use
- Alcohol overuse
- Safe sex protection
- Safe driving habits
- Skin protection
- Mental health issues
- Healthy weight
- Diet
- Exercise

Healthy Life Plan—Milestone 30s

HEALTH PLAN FOR YOUR

30s

Your thirties is a great time to begin cementing your prevention plan. Begin tracking things like weight, blood pressure, and cholesterol. Be aware of pre-diabetes symptoms. Your cancer risk rises in your thirties, so get the screenings you need and watch for symptoms. Women, if you don't have children yet, think about prenatal and reproductive health.

Mission Statement: ______________________________

____

Sample: See my primary care doctor regularly to assess my health risks and manage my weight, blood pressure, and physical activity.

Goal ______________________________

Actions

- ______________
- ______________
- ______________
- ______________
- ______________
- ______________

Goal ______________________________

Actions

- ______________
- ______________
- ______________
- ______________
- ______________
- ______________

Goal ______________________________

Actions

- ______________
- ______________
- ______________
- ______________
- ______________
- ______________

Goal ______________________________

Actions

- ______________
- ______________
- ______________
- ______________
- ______________
- ______________

Goal ______________________________

Actions

- ______________
- ______________
- ______________
- ______________
- ______________
- ______________

Example:

Goal *Establish prevention*

Actions *Find a good doctor*

Get a physical every two years

Review health history

Establish health goals

Prevention and Detection

- Checkup (every two years)
- Dental exam (every year)
- Tetanus booster
- Blood pressure (yearly)
- Cholesterol (every five years)
- Heart health review

Just for women:

- Pap test (every three years)
- Pelvic exam (yearly)
- Breast exam (yearly)

Healthstyle Habits to Consider

- Smoking or tobacco use
- Recreational drug use
- Alcohol overuse
- Safe sex protection
- Safe driving habits
- Skin protection
- Mental health issues
- Stress management
- Healthy weight
- Diet
- Exercise

Healthy Life Plan—Milestone 40s

It's time to really kick your prevention into gear and weed out risky healthstyle habits that are still hitching a ride from your thirties. Be sure you've got a good assessment of your health risks and a plan for getting the screenings and exams you need. Being aware of your family history, watching for any symptoms, and catching them early is also critical.

HEALTH PLAN FOR YOUR

40s

Mission Statement: ______________________________

____

Sample: Get regular screenings and checkups, stay on top of my weight and exercise, and watch out for extra stress.

Goal ______________________________

Actions

- ______________
- ______________
- ______________
- ______________
- ______________

Goal ______________________________

Actions

- ______________
- ______________
- ______________
- ______________
- ______________

Goal ______________________________

Actions

- ______________
- ______________
- ______________
- ______________
- ______________

Goal ______________________________

Actions

- ______________
- ______________
- ______________
- ______________
- ______________

Goal ______________________________

Actions

- ______________
- ______________
- ______________
- ______________
- ______________

Example:

Goal *Stop smoking*

Actions *Talk with doctor*

Explore nicotine aids

Write up goals and plan

Set stop date

Prevention and Detection

- Checkup (every year)
- Dental exam (every year)
- Tetanus booster
- Blood pressure (yearly)
- Cholesterol (every five years)
- Blood sugar test
- Vision and hearing tests
- Skin exam (yearly)
- Heart health review

For women:

- Mammogram (every two years)
- Pap test (every three years)
- Pelvic exam (yearly)

For men:

- Digital rectal exam (yearly)
- Prostate exam

Healthstyle Habits to Consider

- Smoking or tobacco use
- Recreational drug use
- Alcohol overuse
- Safe sex protection
- Safe driving habits
- Skin protection
- Mental health issues
- Stress management
- Healthy weight
- Diet
- Exercise
- Women: calcium intake

Healthy Life Plan—Milestone 50s

Heart health is critical. If you've got weight issues, get them under control. Diabetes risk increases but can be minimized by diet and exercise. Unhealthy habits may begin to show effects. Now's the perfect time to get motivated to change your habits, stay on top of your prevention, and get on course for a long, healthy life with as few health issues as possible.

HEALTH PLAN FOR YOUR

50s

Mission Statement: ____________________

____

Sample: Protect my heart health through diet, exercise, and stress management. Get preventive screenings and stay motivated.

Goal ____________________

Actions

- ________ • ________
- ________ • ________
- ________ • ________

Goal ____________________

Actions

- ________ • ________
- ________ • ________
- ________ • ________

Goal ____________________

Actions

- ________ • ________
- ________ • ________
- ________ • ________

Goal ____________________

Actions

- ________ • ________
- ________ • ________
- ________ • ________

Goal ____________________

Actions

- ________ • ________
- ________ • ________
- ________ • ________

Example:

Goal *Control blood pressure*

Actions *Talk with doctor*

Reduce salt/change diet

Exercise four times weekly

Monitor pressure monthly

Prevention and Detection

- Heart health review
- Checkup (every year)
- Dental exam (every year)
- Tetanus booster
- Blood pressure (yearly)
- Cholesterol (every five years)
- Blood sugar test
- Vision and hearing tests
- Skin exam (yearly)
- Fecal blood occult (yearly)
- Sigmoidoscopy (twice)
- Colonoscopy (once)

For women:

- Mammogram (every year)
- Pap test (every three years)
- Pelvic exam (yearly)
- Menopause treatment

For men:

- Digital rectal exam (yearly)
- Prostate exam
- PSA blood test (yearly)
- Prostatitis diagnosis

Healthstyle Habits to Consider

- Attack any lingering healthstyle habits
- Skin protection
- Mental health issues
- Healthy weight
- Diet and exercise
- Women: calcium intake

Healthy Life Plan—Milestone 60s

Your sixties milestone brings a few new conditions to be on guard for. Stroke risk goes up, so know the symptoms and get treatment early. Bacterial infections also become more of a risk if you're in the hospital more frequently for treatment of any health issues. And don't neglect your healthstyle habits—they're still the key to keeping you feeling great.

HEALTH PLAN FOR YOUR

60s

Mission Statement: ____________________

____

Sample: Understand various symptoms (including stroke, heart attack, cancer) and how to get help. Improve my diet and physical activity.

Goal ____________________

Actions
- ____________
- ____________
- ____________
- ____________
- ____________

Goal ____________________

Actions
- ____________
- ____________
- ____________
- ____________
- ____________

Goal ____________________

Actions
- ____________
- ____________
- ____________
- ____________
- ____________

Goal ____________________

Actions
- ____________
- ____________
- ____________
- ____________
- ____________

Goal ____________________

Actions
- ____________
- ____________
- ____________
- ____________
- ____________

Example:

Goal *Reduce cancer risk*

Actions *Talk with doctor*

Five to six veggies per day

Walk (exercise) daily

Get current on screenings

Prevention and Detection

- Heart health review
- Checkup (every year)
- Dental exam (every year)
- Tetanus booster
- Pneumonia vaccination
- Flu vaccination (yearly)
- Blood pressure (yearly)
- Cholesterol (every five years)
- Blood sugar test
- Vision and hearing tests
- Glaucoma (every two years)
- Skin exam (yearly)
- Fecal blood occult (yearly)
- Sigmoidoscopy (twice)
- Colonoscopy (once)

For women:
- Mammogram (every year)
- Pap test (every three years)
- Pelvic exam (yearly)
- Bone density test

For men:
- Digital rectal exam (yearly)
- Prostate exam
- PSA blood test (yearly)
- Prostatitis diagnosis

Health Conditions to Watch

- Cancer
- Stroke
- Lung disease
- Pneumonia
- Diabetes
- Parkinson's
- Bacterial infections

Healthy Life Plan—Milestone 70+

In your seventies and beyond, protecting both your physical and mental wellness are key. Alzheimer's is an increased risk, so know the symptoms and get treatment as early as possible. You'll also want to watch for injuries to your bones and joints, as the possibility of accidents increases. Don't neglect your vision, hearing, or mental health.

HEALTH PLAN FOR YOUR

70+

Mission Statement: ____________________

____

Sample: Lower my risk of injury, get treatment early for any symptoms, and make sure I have a support system to help with care.

Goal ____________________

Actions

- ____________
- ____________
- ____________
- ____________
- ____________
- ____________

Goal ____________________

Actions

- ____________
- ____________
- ____________
- ____________
- ____________
- ____________

Goal ____________________

Actions

- ____________
- ____________
- ____________
- ____________
- ____________
- ____________

Goal ____________________

Actions

- ____________
- ____________
- ____________
- ____________
- ____________
- ____________

Goal ____________________

Actions

- ____________
- ____________
- ____________
- ____________
- ____________
- ____________

Example:

Goal *Protect my bones*

Actions *Talk with doctor*

Take calcium supplement

Be physically active weekly

Check home for safety

Prevention and Detection

- Safety review
- Vision and hearing tests
- Glaucoma (every two years)
- Checkup (every year)
- Dental exam (every year)
- Tetanus booster
- Flu vaccination (yearly)
- Blood pressure (yearly)
- Cholesterol (every five years)
- Heart health review
- Skin exam (yearly)
- Fecal blood occult (yearly)
- Sigmoidoscopy (every five years)
- Colonoscopy (every ten years)

For women:

- Mammogram (every year)
- Pap test (every three years)
- Pelvic exam (yearly)

For men:

- Digital rectal exam (yearly)
- Prostate exam
- PSA blood test (yearly)

Health Conditions to Watch

- Cancer
- Stroke
- Lung disease
- Pneumonia
- Diabetes
- Parkinson's
- Bacterial infections
- Bone fractures
- Alzheimer's

Taylor's Sixth Law of Health

Your health power is contagious—spread it around.

Prescription 5

Harness Your Power

Conquering the Beast

In December 1995, after a routine physical, Al got the startling news that he had Stage 3 esophageal cancer. His doctor gave him six months to live if he did nothing, twelve to eighteen months if he had surgery to remove the tumor. Merry Christmas. But Al didn't approach this news as many people would. He decided that this wasn't just a disease; it was a Beast that was gunning for a fight. And he was just the guy to give it to him. After his surgery the mirror in his bedroom became a landing place for Post-it notes containing messages from friends, his own thoughts, and quotes to push him forward in his fight. One such note read, "If this cancer is coming after me, it better be ready to deal with someone with an attitude. —Al, Christmas 1995."

> **RESOURCE**
>
> **Find Online Support Groups**
>
> Find a nifty directory of online support groups for a huge selection of health issues at www.dmoz.org/Health/Support_Groups/.

Certainly these weren't the words of a cancer victim. And true to form, Al's surgery successfully eliminated his tumor and all seemed rosy. Then in September 1996, the Beast resurfaced. This time, the battle would require a stronger arsenal, and Al embarked on an aggressive round of chemotherapy and radiation treatments. Friends and e-mail acquaintances gathered through his Internet support group were unsure whether to offer him congratulations or condolences, but true to form, Al never lost faith in his ability to win the war . . .

> We never got close to condolences. The treatment was no picnic. But, as assaultive as it was, I always knew this was just temporary. It was the price of teaching the Beast one more lesson. I never felt so bad that I was tempted to just wallow in despair. I began to embrace the notion that I was a cancer victor rather than a cancer patient. I never did think of myself as a cancer victim.

So what was Al's stealth weapon? Ten years after his victory over the Beast, with no signs of cancer in his body, Al reflects on how the battle was waged.

> I have learned that people who join the [esophageal cancer support] group have a longevity substantially greater than the statistical average. That is not just a statistical anomaly. People who are proactive in the defense of their health do better. They have encouraging family and friends. Their physicians are impressed with their knowledge and determination and pay closer attention. They live their lives more richly even as they endure the assault of treatment. Rather than be debilitated by it, they take energy from their fight with the Beast. Fighters live longer and they live their lives more richly as they fight.
>
> And those who begin sharing the story of their victories—even the tiny milestones on the path to victory—do even better. When I was [diagnosed] the average longevity was nineteen months. What would you say the odds would be that three random people diagnosed within a month of one another would beat the nineteen-month average? What are the odds that they would beat it by double? By triple? Over 100 months ago in the spring of 1995 a retired air force colonel in Texas, a young grandfather software engineer in Wisconsin, and a professional pleasure boater in the San Francisco Bay area were [diagnosed] with [esophageal cancer]. Rather advanced [esophageal cancer] at that—all Stage 3s. Between them there were a couple of

dozen hot lymph nodes. They came together to become the nucleus of the EC [Esophageal Cancer] Group. And Jim, Steve, and myself are all around today. A miracle? Three miracles? Coincidence? Luck? Who cares? But I have come to believe that positive attitudes heal. And mentoring stokes the immune system.

Life is busy. Life is full. Life is rich. Life is sweet. And I am grateful.

Al, EC Victor, 2005

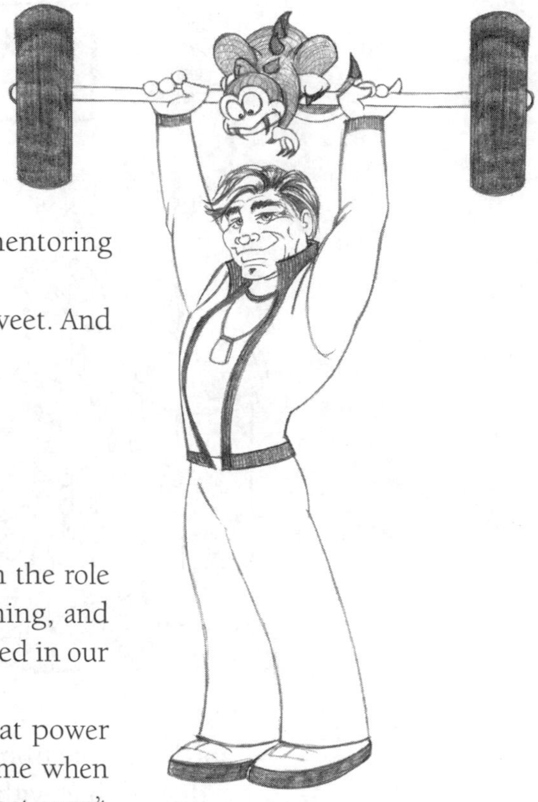

The Kids' Table

The design of our health care system keeps us in the role of a child in our health: powerless, not questioning, and passive—relegated to the kids' table and uninvolved in our own destiny.

But people like Al show that you can grab that power back and demonstrate how strong you can become when you do. Is this just "think positive" sunshine that won't really do you any good? Absolutely not. I'm not talking only about the power of positive thinking. That's powerful in and of itself, and from personal experience I'm a firm believer in the connection between your mental state and your physical well-being. But look closely again at what Al says about the real-life effect your Health Power can have.

> People who are proactive in the defense of their health do better. They have *encouraging family and friends*. Their *physicians* are impressed with their knowledge and determination and *pay closer attention . . . Rather than be debilitated* by it, *they take energy* from their fight with the Beast.

Claiming your Health Power means that those around you will understand that you take your health seriously and they'll take it seriously, too. It means that doctors, nurses, hospital workers, coworkers, your boss, your family, and your friends will get caught up in your enthusiasm about your health. You'll get more respect

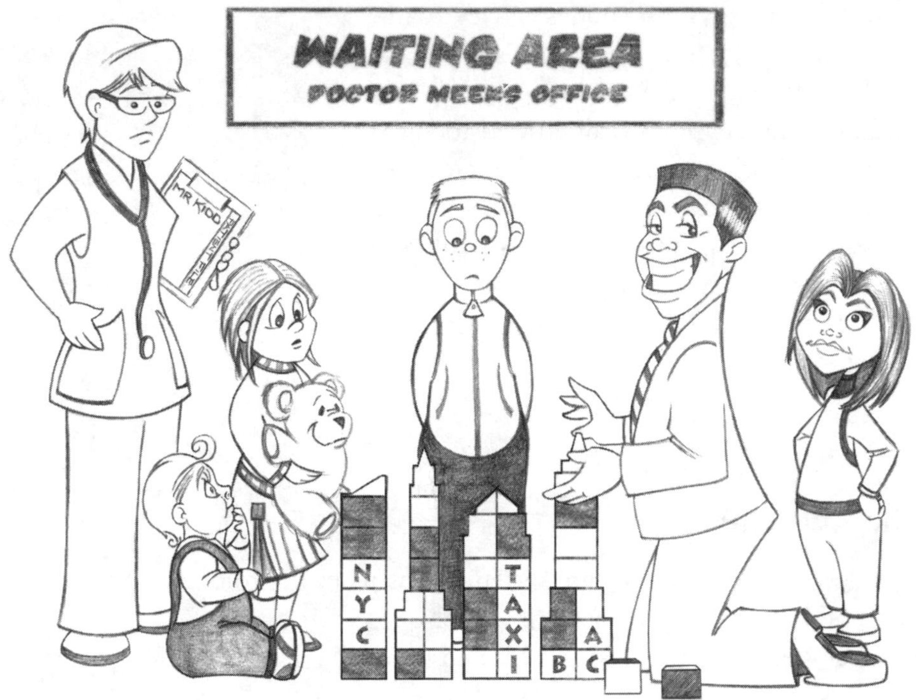

and better care from doctors. You'll infect those around you, not with a disease, but with an excitement about making good healthstyle choices, feeling better, and getting more out of life. By picking up and reading this book, you took an active step toward unleashing that power. It could be that you or someone you love is dealing with one or more health issues. You might just be tired of being left out of your own health care circle. You may even be fed up with all of the nonsense you hear on the news and ready to make your own decisions about your health. Whatever your motivation, you're choosing to become an active partner in your own health.

4 Health Books Everyone Should Own

American Medical Association Family Medical Guide

Johns Hopkins Symptoms and Remedies

Johns Hopkins Consumer's Guide to Drugs

The Complete Guide to Pediatric Symptoms

Ninety-two percent of Americans say they want to be more informed health care consumers, yet over half say they doubt they could make the right choices. We know how important it is to be involved in our own health, but our self-perceptions make us think that we're not really qualified to plan for our health or make important decisions. So often it's just easier to avoid it and hope the doctor will take care of everything for us.

Balance of Power

Do you rely on your health care team too much or too little?	Answer true or false to each statement.	
1. I want my doctors to make most of the important decisions about my health.	T	F
2. My doctors are responsible for whether my treatment works.	T	F
3. I can't control if I get sick.	T	F
4. I trust that the government will make sure that the medications I take are safe.	T	F
5. It is my doctor's responsibility to know everything about my health.	T	F
6. If I have a health condition, my doctors will know which treatment is best.	T	F
7. My doctors should be responsible for keeping me well.	T	F
8. In the hospital, the nurses are responsible for my safety.	T	F
9. My primary care doctor should coordinate my care.	T	F
10. My time is too valuable to waste worrying about my own health.	T	F
11. I will wait to worry about my health until I get older.	T	F
12. I don't want to be in charge of my health.	T	F
13. In the hospital, there are safeguards to protect my health.	T	F
14. I don't understant what I need to do to improve my health.	T	F
15. I am not qualified to make my own health care decisions.	T	F

Scoring and Evaluation

Total Number: True __________ **False** __________

Mostly true:	You may be relying too much on others to make decisions for you. You need to do more to become an active part of your health care.
About the same true as false:	You are taking some responsibility for your own health, but come on, it's your life. Get involved.
Mostly false:	*Great!* You are taking charge of your health. Always consider the opinions of your health care professionals, but remember that you are the one who has to live with the results of any condition or treatment. Stay involved.

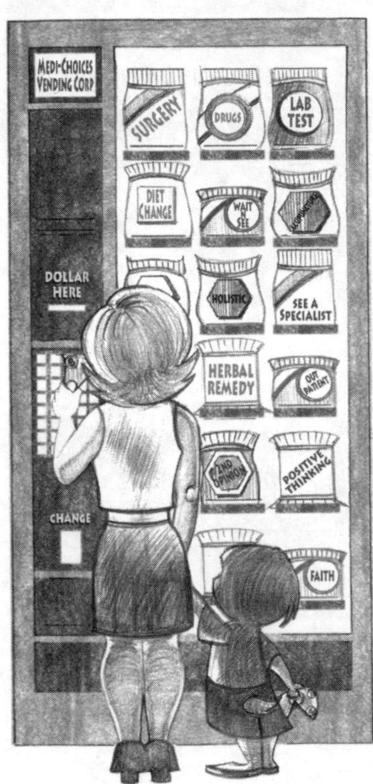

Why do we have so little faith in ourselves? It's not just us. There are many forces at play in keeping us naked on the table—some intentional, some inadvertent. Messages that can undermine your Health Power are all around you.

You Choose, You Lose

Negative messages can come under the pretense of "consumer choice" in a trend I call "You Choose, You Lose." In Barry Schwartz's book *The Paradox of Choice: Why More Is Less*, he not only laments the overabundance of health choices offered up, but often sees these choices as a way for the government, corporations, and the medical community to shirk responsibility. By making us feel that our health issues are a result of our own bad choices, the system lets those who are supposed to keep us healthy and give us healthy products off the hook.

It's not their fault you eat junk food—it's your choice.

It's not their fault that you didn't have the test that could have saved your life—it was your choice.

It's not their fault that a drug caused side effects—it was your choice.

Consider this letter from a marketing executive that appeared in a weekly magazine about advertising. It was sent in response to an editorial about the skyrocketing rate of obesity in American children.

> Only in America do we blame obesity on marketing efforts. This type of fingerpointing only happens when the majority of society does not want to take responsibility for their own actions. Instead of blaming marketing efforts for obese and unhealthy children, lawyers, consumer groups and government agencies should look at the real underlining [*sic*] issues causing obesity in children: boredom, laziness, no supervision from parents and unhealthy eating habits are the main attributes to obesity. It does not have much to do with marketing unhealthy junk-food items. . . . Instead of blaming the companies' marketing message we should blame parents who let their children eat what ever [*sic*] their hearts desire, children for being couch potatoes and video-game junkies and parents and children for

not being more creative at finding hobbies and activities that will keep everyone healthy and active.

This just begs the question: If marketing to children doesn't make them eat junk food, why does the food industry spend $15 billion (yes, that's *billion*) on advertising every year doing just that? This letter shows the opinion of just one person, but it's amazing that someone is blaming children for actually responding to the more than fifty-eight advertising messages that they see every day.

It's mixed messages like these that help foster our feelings of inadequacy and blame. We've heard so often that sickness is our fault, we immediately look to blame ourselves. Of course we don't feel qualified to manage our own health—look at what a mess we've made of things. We're overweight; we have skyrocketing rates of diabetes, heart disease, and high blood pressure; we don't get any exercise; we eat badly; and we don't take care of ourselves. Well, I think that's just a bunch of baloney.

Do we sometimes make questionable choices? Of course. But we also know more about our health than we ever have and have waged some pretty impressive battles against threats to our health. The folks I see on my travels around the country have what I call a Healthy Spirit—they want to be more informed about their health so they can make good healthstyle choices, are determined to live their lives to the fullest, and want to do everything they can to protect their health and the health of those they love.

RESOURCE

Is the Food You're Eating Safe?

Check out food recalls by calling 888-463-6332 or click on www.fda.gov.

Not Just Words and Images

Every day you see and hear dozens of messages, both internal and external, that frame how you think about your health. Some are as simple as the language used to describe patients and their conditions—"the patient complains of . . ." makes us sound like whiny, sniveling children; "Ms. Kaufman suffers from . . ." implies a passive victim, rather than someone with a condition she wants to treat and manage. It may seem insignificant, but don't underestimate how words and phrases can make you feel about your health. Words are powerful. They tell us how to feel and reinforce incredibly powerful thoughts and perceptions. They become so commonplace that you and your doctors don't even stop to think about the negative message these words send.

Doc Talk

Doctors and health officials have struggled throughout history to describe patients who don't do what they're told (how dare they!). Here are some examples of the "wonderful" names that have been given to patients:

From the 1890s to the 1940s the language used to describe tuberculosis patients who did not follow treatment instructions included *ignorant, vicious, recalcitrant*, and *defaulters*.

Before 1960, *faithless* became popular for referring to patients who did not follow recommended treatments. *Untrustworthy* and *unreliable* were also used.

From the 1970s and up to today, *noncompliant* and *nonadherent* have been widely used. They are going out of style because of the implication that treatment is dictated by the doctor, rather than developed together with the patient.

Once you are diagnosed with a medical condition, you get slapped with a label, as if you stop being a person and become a disease. You're no longer Martin Kramer, father, business owner, and expert on model airplanes but become instead Martin Kramer, diabetic. The person you are is lost, condensed down to that one little word. No one wants to be known by their medical conditions. Let's stop calling people diabetic, asthmatic, or arthritic, and let's call us what we are—people with conditions that need to be treated and managed.

Anyone who's been in the hospital knows what it's like to be made to sit in a crowded waiting room in a gown with those paper slippers on your feet, waiting to be called in for your test. That bracelet they put around your wrist that you can't take off without a blowtorch with your patient number on it is appropriate, because in many ways that's how you're treated—like a number. You become a nameless, faceless patient—not a person.

I remember a few years back when a simple test I had came back "abnormal" for some cancerous cells. "Probably nothing," my doctor said, but then sent me to one of the leading cancer centers in the world, which happened to be down the street, to have some additional tests. I'm not saying they weren't nice—they were. Everyone was unbelievably sensitive, maybe a little too sensitive. Before going, I hadn't been worried at all. My doctor said the chances were extremely remote because I was young and had absolutely no symptoms. But the staff at the hospital treated me as if I had already been diagnosed, with pained looks of concern on their faces. And the minute I put on a gown and was made to be wheeled to the exam room, I really began to feel as if I was sick. "I can walk!" I wanted to scream, but felt that would probably be considered impolite. And they were just trying to be nice. I don't think health professionals mean to treat you as if you're sick, but I also believe they don't realize how subtle some of these messages are and how undermining they can be to your Healthy Spirit.

It's not just the words; it's the images, too. Jake Harwood, an associate professor of communications at the University of Arizona and an expert on the ways language helps define group identities, has conducted research that shows it's nearly impossible to find images of older adults that don't involve the assumption that they are unhealthy. Mr. Harwood found that older folks are depicted as declining both mentally and physically, particularly in advertising. Ads featuring models in their fifties and sixties are almost exclusively for health products, often tagged with a subtle threat. "If you don't use our medicine," Mr. Harwood relates, "you won't be able to have fun with your grandchildren. . . . There's a positive portrayal, but it's grounded in that script of aging and decline." Mr. Harwood told me he believes this sends the message that growing older equals bad health. "The obsessive linking of old age and ill health in the media make it very difficult for the average person to think about other aspects of aging or to consider the positive elements of aging—those get totally lost." Likewise, he's found that health just isn't talked about a lot in our culture for younger adults, "except perhaps in the context of things like STDs, drug use, etc.—also stereotypical in their own way. Apart from that, it doesn't seem to be discussed a lot, even though it's tremendously important. Ads for health-related products pretty much have no young people in them."

Pop Quiz! Mental Health

1. Fifty percent of American adults have a mental health condition. True False
2. The most common mental condition is depression. True False
3. People with schizophrenia have multiple personalities. True False
4. Prisons house more people with mental health conditions than any other institution. True False
5. Cat owners have a higher rate of psychiatric disorders than non–cat owners. True False

Answers

1. False. The figure is closer to 22 percent.
2. False. Anxiety is the most common. Depression is second.
3. False. This misconception comes from the symptom of hearing voices.
4. True. Three out of ten prisoners receive mental health treatment.
5. False. Cat owners actually have fewer mental health conditions.

Healthy Spirit, Healthy Body

Along with the external messages you see and hear every day, your own internal messages can sabotage your Healthy Spirit from the inside out, keeping you from using your Health Power to take charge of your health and feel better. You may feel you're not capable or ready to manage your health or make the right decisions. You may

Know Way!

You can't catch a cold at the North Pole in the winter. Ironically, cold germs can't survive in the extremely cold temperatures.

feel that being diagnosed with a health condition will make your life miserable and prefer to bury your head in the sand. Since being healthy is one of the keys to being happy, many of us assume that once you've been diagnosed with a health condition, your life as you know it will cease to exist. Take Brian, for example.

Brian was one of the most dynamic young men you'd ever want to know. Naturally funny and charismatic, Brian started his career working in a large corporation, but had gotten burned out by what he called "cubicle life" and was excited to be working at our small company where he could really make an impact. A strong, healthy, twenty-four-year-old, Brian considered himself a fitness nut, although, typically for his age, he didn't seem to give too much thought to his overall health. I started to notice a difference in Brian over a period of about three weeks. Normally beating me to the office (which isn't hard to do), Brian started showing up late and calling in sick. And when he was there, he just wasn't himself. When I'd ask him if everything was okay, he'd say, "I don't know, I just haven't been feeling well. I seem to have this flu that I can't shake." My suggestions for Brian to see his doctor were brushed off with "I just need to get some rest." Finally, one day, Brian came into my office nearly in tears. "I think I have to go," he said.

"Where?" I asked, thinking he was leaving the company for another job.

"To the doctor," Brian told me. "I just can't seem to shake this feeling and I'm losing weight, too. I'm scared."

We talked about his symptoms, how he'd been feeling, and what he would say to his doctor.

I was relieved that he'd finally decided it was time to get a professional opinion. The next day, Brian called to give me the news. He was in the hospital and had been diagnosed with type 1 diabetes. His blood sugar level had been so dangerously high that he had almost died. He would have to take insulin the rest of his life. He seemed shell-shocked, not understanding where this condition had come from. Brian returned to work a couple of weeks later and seemed to be in better spirits than he'd been in a long time. Knowing that Brian would have emotional ups and downs, we all tried to give him the support and space he needed to cope with his new reality. Then one day I popped into his office to discuss a new project to find Brian sitting at his desk in tears. He'd been to our health library and his desk was piled high with textbooks on diabetes.

"I'm so depressed," he said. "I just want my old life back. These books say so many horrible things about having diabetes. I'm going to die ten years sooner. I'm going to go blind or have an amputation. I'm going to be impotent. What if I have kids, are they going to have diabetes, too?"

I leaned over and moved the books to the floor. "Brian," I said, "it's completely natural to feel overwhelmed. You've been handed a *huge* challenge that you never expected. I'd be worried about you if you weren't stressed out. But let's stop looking at what's been taken from you and look at what you have. You're a healthy, strong, twenty-four-year-old guy."

Brian snickered, "Oh yeah, real healthy."

"You're wrong," I said. "Now is when your healthy habits are going to pay off. You're not unhealthy. You've got diabetes. Your pancreas doesn't function like a normal pancreas. That's not an illness—it's a condition that you have to manage. Yes, there are downsides that can happen if you don't take care of yourself. Yes, you're going to have to change your habits and think about your health more, but the upside is that you're going to have an awareness of your health that other people your age just don't have. I'm not giving you some look-on-the-sunny-side line, because it does stink. But it's gonna stink whether you take charge of it or not—and it will stink less if you do. I'm just telling you that with the support of friends, family, and doctors, you can take control of this and live a long, healthy life—unless of course you get hit by a bus tomorrow!"

Brian had been thrown in the deep end. In an instant, his self-perception had changed from a carefree, average young male to someone with real health issues and concerns. Brian could either

Know When to Go to the ER

Each situation is different, so use this only as a general guide. If you have doubts about your condition, call 9-1-1 or go to the emergency room. Go to the ER if you have:

- Broken bones
- Serious cut, burn, or wound
- Severe, persistent vomiting
- Severe, persistent diarrhea
- Severe pain
- Nosebleed after head injury
- Coughed up blood
- Persistent dizziness/fainting
- Fever over 104 degrees
- Abdominal pain from an injury
- Abdominal pain with high fever
- Abdominal pain with vaginal bleeding
- Severe bleeding in pregnancy
- Severe depression, anxiety, or panic
- Sudden, persistent pain in testicles
- Fever in children (rectal)
  - Over 100.2 degrees (under 3 months)
  - Over 102 degrees (3–6 months)
  - Over 104 degrees (under 14 years)

5 minute clinic: 4 Ways We Sabotage Our Thoughts

Negative thoughts can be hard to overcome, especially when it comes to your health. See if you fall victim to any of these subtle sabotage techniques.

1. **Focusing on the negative.** This is often called "filtering" by psychologists because you "filter out" all of the positive and see only the negative. If you are diagnosed with a condition, you may hear only the negative statistics and outcomes.
   Strategy: Instead of putting yourself on the negative side, switch to the positive. Find out what steps and treatments people who have a positive outcome take. Be one of them.
2. **Taking it personally.** When something bad happens, you immediately think that it's your fault or has to do with you. If your child gets the flu, you think it's because you didn't dress him warmly enough for school.
   Strategy: Accept that things happen that are outside your control. Minimize your risks and move forward.
3. **Anticipating the worst.** You automatically believe the worst will happen. If you are diagnosed with a condition, you immediately ask how long you've got rather than focus on treatments and cures.
   Strategy: Nobody wants you to ignore all possible outcomes, but don't get distracted from positive steps by focusing only on the dire consequences.
4. **Seeing black and white.** Do you feel you have to be perfect or else you're a failure? In health, there's a lot more middle ground. A diagnosis is just the first step in solving a problem and getting to your healthiest life.
   Strategy: Just because you've been diagnosed with a health condition doesn't mean your life is ruined. Find the way to live your best life.

choose to reframe his thinking and take charge of his health or remain a child, seemingly powerless against this "disease."

Research shows that even serious health conditions do not have to impact your Healthy Spirit as negatively as you might think. In a recent clinical study, PDAs (Personal Digital Assistants—like Palm Pilots) were given to a group of people who were receiving dialysis treatment for their kidneys three times a week as well as to a group of people not managing a chronic condition. The PDAs prompted them to answer questions at random times throughout the day about their mood, emotions, pain, energy level, and overall life satisfaction. The researchers found no real difference between the answers of the people who were receiving dialysis and those who were not. Not surprisingly, the people in the study who were not on dialysis wrongly predicted that they would be much unhappier if they were in the shoes of the dialysis patients. It suggests that the depression often found in people who have just been diagnosed with a health condition could be partly because they assume that having the condition will be far worse than it is. In reality, it seems that we can adapt to managing a health condition more easily than we think.

And a growing body of research is demonstrating that having a Healthy Spirit is important not just to your health, but to your life. One study conducted on older adults showed a direct link between how they rated their health and how long they lived! Study participants who gave their health a "bad/poor" or "fair" grade were more than twice as likely to die within four years as those who rated themselves "excellent." Of course, some of these results may have to do with the people in the study actually having health issues, accounting both for their negative self-assessment and shortened life span. But the study also revealed that not only did these self-perceptions often predict mortality, the people who rated themselves as healthier took more control and did more to improve their health and well-being.

As in other parts of your life, health becomes a self-fulfilling prophecy. If you think of yourself as healthy, you'll take steps to make that perception come true. That's why it's important to explore your health perceptions and use tactics that will help you feel more in control of your health and exercise your Health Power to live longer and feel better.

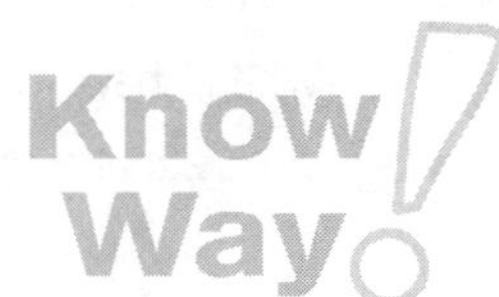

Discovered on a remote island, the dodo bird became extinct in 1681 because it had no natural fear of man and could not adapt to being hunted.

Optimism Inventory

A positive attitude can help you in many aspects of life, but can it actually keep you healthy? Research tells us "yes," it can. People with self-confidence and optimism have an easier time overcoming pain and adversity and typically have better medical outcomes. Researchers at Yale found that people with a good outlook live seven and a half years longer than their gloomier counterparts. Answer each question as truthfully as you can and read the Positivity tips at right.

1. When I look in the mirror, I see . . .
   a. a person who is attractive, self-confident, and in control.
   b. a person who is average and a little bit unsure of himself.
   c. a person who is unattractive and doesn't have it together.

Everyone has something uniquely special. Focus on your positive qualities and strengths, not the negative.

(continued)

Optimism Inventory (continued)

2. When I have a problem, I tend to . . . a. look for someone or something to blame—it's not my fault. b. complain to anyone who will listen, but don't do much to fix it. c. take responsibility for the problem and focus on the solution.	Taking responsibility will help you see problems as mere challenges to be overcome and move on to solving them.
3. My overall outlook on life is usually . . . a. sunny and optimistic. I'm definitely a glass-half-full person. b. trying to find the good in people but often getting disappointed. c. pessimistic and negative. I rarely see people doing good things.	Make a list of the positive things and people in your life and try to shift your focus away from the negative.
4. When I have to make a decision, I tend to . . . a. agonize over it and ask someone else to make it for me. b. ask everyone I know what they think and then try to figure it out. c. evaluate the options and then make my own decision.	Getting the advice of others can be helpful, but you are best qualified to judge what is right for you.
5. When I have an important task to do, I usually . . . a. attack the task and get it done right away. b. proceed to do it, but get easily distracted by something else. c. procrastinate until I have to get it done.	Procrastination tends to elevate levels of stress and frustration. Instead, develop a plan and get moving!
6. When I make a mistake, I typically . . . a. crawl under the covers feeling embarrassed and ashamed. b. figure it is someone else's fault, and hope no one notices. c. know everyone makes mistakes and I am no different. I take responsibility and try to fix it.	It's normal to be embarrassed by a mistake, but don't blow it out of proportion. Do what you can to fix it and move on.
7. When that little voice in my head talks, I usually hear . . . a. confident tips on how I can approach a situation positively. b. supportive statements reminding me of my limitations. c. critical and negative statements that put me in my place.	Negative thoughts take away our power by scaring us that we will fail. Give yourself positive affirmations and stop those negative thoughts now!
8. When people give me feedback or criticism, I . . . a. take it personally. I'm sure they're right. b. snap right back at them with something equally critical. c. appreciate it but keep it in perspective.	Giving too much weight to the views of others can minimize your own feelings and self-confidence. Keep their motivations and outlook in mind.

The Eventual Patient

We're all *eventual patients*, because someday we'll all become patients, one way or another. How you harness your Health Power will determine the kind of care you get, the quality of your life, and sometimes even if you live or die. That's why you can choose to claim your Health Power now, when the choice is yours, or like Brian, when a health event occurs that shocks you into awareness. You can stay stuck in the framework of the ten-year-old, sitting on the table in that little paper gown, powerless, waiting for the big doctor to come through the door, or you can harness your Health Power, make choices about your life, and guide your own health and destiny.

Take a look at the 5 Steps to Changing Your Own Negative Messages. It will take a little practice to make changing negative thoughts to positive ones a regular habit. The key is to catch the negative thoughts before they have a chance to cloud your thinking or your actions. Once you've done that, you can switch or "reframe" the negative words to positive thoughts.

Your thoughts and perceptions about your health can give you the strength to take charge or can turn you into an Ostrich (see chapter 1). As you become aware of the negative messages you see and hear, you can make the decision to reframe how you think about your health. When you do, you'll be amazed at how easy it will be to reclaim your Healthy Spirit and take control. You'll feel stronger and better about your health every day, and you'll be ready to face your health challenges with a positive outlook and the power to fight.

5 Steps to Changing Your Own Negative Messages

1. Pay attention to your inner voice.
2. Listen for negative words.
3. Stop using the negative words.
4. Switch the negative word to a positive one.
5. Reframe the negative statement into a positive action statement.

Healthy Spirit Exploration Exercise

Here's an exercise that will help you begin to clear out those negative messages and reframe your thoughts in a more positive spirit. Take a few moments to consider your perceptions about health—your own health, your family's health, medical conditions, treatments, and so on. Then read each statement below. For each negative statement, write your own positive spin. I've done the first couple for you as examples.

1. I am not qualified to make medical decisions.
Positive Spin

My doctor is an important resource in my Healthy Life Plan, but only I know what I want from my health, what's important to me, and what I'm willing to do and not do to be healthy.

2. Everyone gets sick. It's only a matter of time.
Positive Spin

I know that I may get a health condition, but I will do what I can to stay healthy and make good choices. If I do get a condition, I will get smart about the condition, get the treatment that is right for me, and manage the condition so that I can live a long, full life.

3. Sick people are weak.
Positive Spin

4. I don't have the time to worry about my health.
Positive Spin

RESOURCE

Self-Esteem Games Online

Try out some cool games designed to help you reach positivity at www.selfesteemgames.mcgill.ca.

5. My health problems are my own fault.
Positive Spin

6. Somebody else should worry about my health.
Positive Spin

Now, write down some of your own negative health messages and reframe them with your own positive spin.

Negative Perception

____

____

Positive Spin

____

____

____

Negative Perception

____

____

Positive Spin

____

____

____

Negative Perception

____

____

Positive Spin

____

____

____

Health Sabotage: Could You Be a Victim?

Researchers say that sabotage from friends and family is one of the primary reasons people can't lose weight or put it back on once they've lost it. And diet isn't the only way those around you may keep you from being your healthiest. Most people don't do it on purpose; it's just that when someone around them begins to change, it may threaten their self-perception. You might make them more aware of their own not-so-healthy habits and make them feel bad that *they're* not doing anything to improve. Take this quiz to see if you could be a victim of health sabotage! Answer true or false for each statement.

My family, friends, and coworkers have poor healthstyle habits. **T F**

It can be extremely hard to try and change your habits when people around you have habits that aren't healthy. For example, people who want to give up smoking have a much better success rate when their spouse gives it up as well. You can't always change everyone around you, so just be aware that you may face temptation.

People in my circle belittle my goals. **T F**

Do the people around you make you feel as if you're silly or deluded for trying to improve your healthstyle habits? It may be less obvious than that—does someone in your office give you articles on why your diet plan won't work or tell you terrible tales about his brother-in-law with the same health condition? Just remember that you are the one who has the ultimate control of how healthy your life can be.

When I change my habits, those around me seem angry or bothered. **T F**

This is a subtle form of sabotage that you might run into. You won't quite understand why, but you'll just get a feeling as if you've done something wrong. "Don't even bother telling Suzy about the birthday party—she doesn't eat cake anyway." But don't let these negative messages get in your way. Go to the party anyway and let everyone see that eating cake isn't the only way to have fun. Give them time and they'll come around.

If I reach my goal, my group of supporters shuts me out. **T F**

If you've got a group you rely on for support, either formal or just a bunch of friends, you might find that if you successfully reach your goal or make your change, your support group makes you feel as if you don't belong. And in a way you don't. They're still struggling with their issues and you've moved on to maintenance. Instead, talk with them openly about it and make them see how valuable you can be as a shining example of success!

My family and friends say that they shouldn't have to change for me. T F

In a way they're right. Nobody has to change their habits for anyone else—it's all about individual choice. And you're going to have to get used to the fact that you need to be able to stick with your changes even though your path is strewn with temptation, bad examples, and others with unhealthy habits. But if you give people time to get over their initial feelings of resentment and see how much better you feel, you'll act as a big motivator. And make sure you don't sabotage others by throwing your change in their face. Always be a source of encouragement, support, and positive reinforcement!

The Circle of Positivity

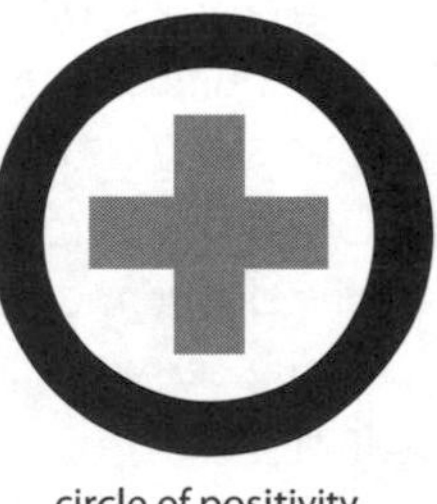
circle of positivity

Okay, I admit it. "Circle of Positivity" sounds corny, but bear with me. A few years back, I began to feel very negative. In talking to people about getting the message of Health Power out to consumers, I got responses like, "Nobody really cares about their health that much," or "People are too lazy to do what it takes to be healthier." Now, this wasn't what I was experiencing. Whenever I spoke at a conference, did call-in radio interviews, or went on book tours, people seemed to love to talk about their health. I've heard hundreds of stories about mystery conditions that eluded diagnosis, how tough it is to help older parents manage medications, or miraculous results from simply changing a child's diet. People I'd met were enormously interested in learning more about how to be healthy and finding out what they could do to be more proactive, and loved to talk about doing more to manage their health and feel better. But then I would come home and go back into meetings with businesspeople and get the same old negative response. It was as if I had two different circles of support, almost two different lives. When I was out with real people, I was excited, upbeat, and had almost endless energy for living life. When I was surrounded by negative people who seemed to always tell me why things couldn't be done and how "dumb" consumers were, I just felt as if I was drowning in negativity. It was changing me as a person—I was just becoming more and more negative. This was not who I wanted to be, but it's hard when you're constantly running into those negative responses—it wears you down. Relating this to my husband one evening, I suddenly blurted out, "I'm going to create a Circle of Positivity around me and there is no longer going to be room for those negative people. I don't dislike them or think less of them—they have their jobs to do. But when I run into one of them, I'm going to move on. They have their opinion, their way of thinking, and I have mine. I'm going to build up my circle with positive people who support what I'm doing and give them my support back." I told you it sounded corny, and trust me, my husband is one of the more cynical people I know. I was expecting a gale of laughter (and another comment on my Suzy Sunshine personality). My husband, instead, stared at me thoughtfully for a few minutes, then said, "You're absolutely right." And I kid you not, from that night on my life began to change. I didn't kick those people out of my life and I didn't treat them any less respectfully when I encountered them in a professional situation. I just didn't give them the gravity I had before—they weren't part of my circle.

I also started to selectively add the right people to my Circle of Positivity. What started out small became a strong circle of support: an encouraging agent, a publisher who cared about quality work, business partners with a high level of integrity and ethics, friends and family who not only gave help but felt free to ask for help when they needed it. I can't imagine going it alone, and neither should you.

You can't manage your health alone, even when you're healthy. You need positive people around you whom you can turn to for information and support and to nurture your Health Power. People who are discouraging or negative will steal your energy, reinforce those negative messages, and sabotage your Healthy Spirit.

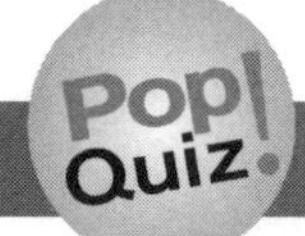

Sexual Health

1. Every day, sexual acts result in 910,000 pregnancies.	True	False
2. The number-one cause of male sterility is bicycle riding.	True	False
3. Eighty-five percent of men who die from a heart attack during sex were cheating on their wives.	True	False
4. The birth control pill can protect you from some sexually transmitted diseases.	True	False
5. Chlamydia, the most common sexually-transmitted disease (STD), is incurable.	True	False

Answers

1. True. So be careful out there.
2. False. The STD chlamydia is. So be careful out there.
3. True. So be careful out there.
4. False. The pill doesn't offer any protection from STDs.
5. False. It can be cured with antibiotics, but it's important to get tested and treated as soon as possible.

Your circle should be as much about giving as it is about getting. The key to building a strong Circle of Positivity is to connect with people who will join you in claiming your Health Power and engage you in supporting theirs as well. Think about including people from each of the following groups as you build your circle.

Doctors and Health Care Professionals

Well-qualified, supportive, and caring doctors will be one of the strongest core groups in your Circle. In the next chapter we're going to look in detail at how to find doctors who are right for you. You'll want to make sure they're professionals whom you trust and respect (and who deserve that respect), whom you feel comfortable with, and who will support you in your desire to manage your health and feel better. You'll also want to find physician's assistants, nurses, and even medical office staff who can contribute to your care. These professionals will be an excellent source of information, motivation,

say no to negativity

5 minute clinic

10 Best Self-Help Books

By no means complete, but here are some of the classics.

1. ***The 7 Habits of Highly Effective People*** by Stephen Covey. Strategies to achieve success in both your personal and professional endeavors.
2. ***Ten Days to Self-Esteem*** by David Burns. Exercises to help you discover why you have negative feelings and how to overcome them.
3. ***The Art of Happiness: A Handbook for Life*** by the Dalai Lama and Howard Cutler. How to find inner peace to defeat depression, anxiety, anger, and jealousy and achieve happiness.
4. ***Don't Sweat the Small Stuff*** by Richard Carlson. One hundred meditations to help keep your emotions in perspective and cherish others.
5. ***How to Win Friends and Influence People*** by Dale Carnegie. The grandfather of people-skills books; teaches you to make others feel important and appreciated.
6. ***Life Strategies*** by Phil McGraw. Accept that you are personally accountable for every element of your life to reach your goals.
7. ***Men Are from Mars, Women Are from Venus*** by John Gray. Acknowledge and accept the differences between men and women to improve your personal relationships.
8. ***The Power of Positive Thinking*** by Norman Vincent Peale. How to have faith in yourself to make good things happen to you.
9. ***Think and Grow Rich*** by Napoleon Hill. "Whatever the mind can conceive and believe, the mind can achieve."
10. ***Who Moved My Cheese?*** by Spencer Johnson. Two mice in a maze show you how to embrace change in your life.

and guidance on keeping you healthy and helping you treat and manage health conditions. If you are managing a specific health condition like diabetes or heart disease, be sure to seek out specialists and experts in that field to provide you with the support you need to live well with your condition.

Health Buddy

Consider adding a Health Buddy to your circle. Whether it's your spouse, a sister or a brother, a neighbor or a colleague, someone who will goose you into sticking with your Healthy Life Plan can help you reach your goals. It's not something we're used to doing, but scheduling a doctor's appointment together is a great way of making sure you go and enjoying your time together while you're there. Why should appointments to protect our health be so grim and serious? The actress Sandra Bullock and her sister, whose mother died from cancer, scheduled an appointment for their first colonoscopies together and even embarked on a shopping spree afterward. Whether it's going for a walk together, calling each other to talk about what you ate today, or just having someone to turn to when you're worried or uptight, your Health Buddy can offer you support and join in your enthusiasm.

My Health Buddy and I take turns keeping each other motivated. We often marvel that we never seem to both be "down" on the same day. When one of us says, "Aw, forget it—I give up," the other one is there to give the needed pep talk. Then come tomorrow it seems the tables turn and the one who was giving the pep talk needs one of her own! Getting discouraged alone is easy. Getting discouraged together is nearly impossible!

Mental Health Professionals

Just as you should have a doctor to help guide your physical well-being, it can be important to have a professional to support your emotional well-being,

How to Find a Therapist

Questions to Ask a Potential Therapist

Before you begin treatment with a mental health professional, interview several to make sure their therapy and professional style are what you want. Here are a few suggestions every therapist should be happy to answer.

1. What is your background—training, education, experience?
2. How long have you been licensed? By which organization?
3. How many clients have you seen with issues similar to mine?
4. What type of therapy approaches do you use?
5. Do you have a treatment agreement that outlines fees, appointments, confidentiality, termination, and so on?

Then ask yourself:

- Am I comfortable with this therapist and his approach?
- Would I like to come back and see him on a regular basis?
- Do I believe his approach would work to make my life better?

especially if you're managing a health condition. It's a great idea to find a mental health professional—whether a psychologist, a family therapist, or a counselor—as a resource you can use if you hit a rough patch or even just as an everyday sounding board. Sometimes it's tough to really see yourself and your own behaviors. Although family and friends often try to be helpful, they may have their own agendas, which can cloud their advice. It's helpful to have an objective, outside view of your challenges, problems, and joys to help you get a clearer picture and improve your focus. To find a good therapist, you can ask your doctor for a recommendation or get ideas from a friend who has had a good experience. You can also get lists from professional organizations or your health insurance plan. It's a good idea to come up with a list of five to six candidates and then call them to make appointments for an interview. Therapy will be much more effective if you find someone you are comfortable with and respect.

RESOURCE

Find a Therapist

For a comprehensive listing of psychiatrists, psychologists, therapists, and counselors, go to www.psychologytoday.com and click on Find a Therapist.

Family, Colleagues, and Friends

This group contains the most important people in your circle, but it can be a challenge to fill. These are the people who surround you every day. We know that you make most of your health decisions, not in the doctor's office but in your everyday life. Your family, friends, and colleagues influence those decisions in a big way. They are the people you spend the most time with and have the most emotional buy-in to. From what you eat to how much physical activity you get, from determining your stress level to keeping up with prevention and treatment, your family members, colleagues, and friends are an important influence on the choices you make. And these are the people you will need help, encouragement, and support from in facing any health challenges that come up.

What's makes it difficult sometimes for your family members and friends is that they are used to you the way you are. People are often uncomfortable with change. Your newfound Health Power may scare or intimidate them. They may not understand why you've got a new outlook on the way you live your life. They may also feel left behind or may be resistant to changing their own habits.

Remember, the key isn't to exclude people from your Circle of Positivity. It's to find those people who will be a positive influence. Start slowly and find ways you can include those around you—start a lunch walking group at work, take your mom on a healthy shopping trip to the grocery store, ask your best friend to go to a diabetes seminar with you. As others see the changes you're making and the positive effect they're having on your life and your health, it won't take long for others to want to get into that circle.

Health Support Pros

From nutritionists to physical therapists, pharmacists and massage therapists, health support professionals form an important part of your circle. Doctors are busy and usually don't have the time to lay out complex treatment or diet plans, answer in-depth questions, or provide the ongoing support you want. A solid stable of health support folks can be worth their weight in gold to help you reach your Healthy Life Plan goals. For example, if you are managing diabetes, a dietitian or a nutritionist who is experienced in diabetes can work with you to come up with a realistic eating plan and help you understand how what and when you eat may affect how you feel. When I was a teenager I was diagnosed with scoliosis, a curvature of the spine. My physical therapist spent two hours showing me how the condition affected my back, coached me in exercises I could do to relieve the strain, and even gave me safety tips on how to take care of my back as I grew older—how to lift objects and carry groceries, and how ballet classes could help my posture—lessons that have stuck with me throughout my life.

Ask your doctor for health support professionals she recommends or talk with family and friends about people they've been to and trust. Also, your health insurance company might have a directory of health support professionals available free of charge or at a reduced rate. Health insurance plans often encourage use of these services since they can provide great support and advice without charging the higher rates of doctors and specialists.

How to Tell Family and Friends You're Worried about Their Health

Telling someone you care about that you're worried about his health can be touchy. He often will react with defensiveness, anger, and denial. Here are some tips for approaching the subject as sensitively as possible:

- Choose the right time.
- Get information about the issue.
- Tell him how you feel about his condition.
- Don't judge him.
- Help him get help.
- Let him know you understand his anger but that your support is unwavering.

Experts and Gurus

Don't limit your circle just to people you have a personal relationship with. The technology of the Internet has brought thousands of experts in their fields right to your doorstep, or more appropriately, right to your computer screen. See a doctor on television with an interesting theory on a condition you're managing? Look her up on the Internet to see if you can send an e-mail. Read a book about a new health theory, and have something you'd like to ask? E-mail the author. You'll be surprised at how often you'll get a response.

Many experts, authors, physicians, and other health professionals have Web sites where they solicit comments, questions, and stories. Look for people you respect and can turn to as another valuable resource. But don't start up a dialogue just to chat. Be sure your question is within their area of expertise. And don't ask someone to make a medical diagnosis over the Internet. Any health professional worth their salt knows that is irresponsible and will most likely direct you back to your physician. If someone does respond with a diagnosis or treatment plan, it's not something you should rely on.

Be cautious getting health information from commercial Web sites that are trying to sell you something. Many offer valuable

Evaluating Health Web Sites

Caveat Lector (Let the reader beware.)

The Internet is a vast source of health information, but not all sites offer accuracy or unbiased sources. Here are some tips to help you get good information. Always remember that free advice is often worth exactly what you pay for it.

1. Know who's behind the site and make sure any sponsors are clearly identified.
2. Look and see when the site has last been updated to make sure the information is current.
3. Check to see if the links are still active.
4. *Always* verify your information with another source, preferably with your doctor, a written source, or at least on another site.

Is This Expert Worthy?

Everyone has a theory for how you can be healthier. Who can you trust, and who's a putz? Here are some tips to help you figure it out.

- He tries to sell you on his "miracle cure." *Putz*
- He examines the pros and cons of various treatments and gives you advice on which one might work best for you. *Trust*
- She says that there is no value in modern medicine. *Putz*
- She explores all aspects of healing, including traditional medicine and natural remedies, as part of an overall plan to treat a condition and keep you healthy. *Trust*

products and services, but many others are just hawking the latest quack cure. Communicating with them may open you up to hundreds of e-mails selling you gimmicks, remedies, and treatments, rather than giving you valid information on your condition. Also, think hard before signing up for a pay subscription service. Some are great and give you access to important health news and help managing your health, but make sure you know exactly what you're signing up for, how much it will really cost you (you don't want to wind up with a monthly charge on your credit card you weren't expecting), and what you're going to get out of it to make sure it's not a scam.

If you don't have access to the Internet or are uncomfortable communicating on the computer, try writing a letter to make contact with an expert. Letters take a little more effort on your part and on the part of the expert you're trying to reach, but they show that you've got a serious question and will usually get a response.

Support Groups

Doctors, family members, friends, and health professionals can all give you important support and advice, but often there is nothing better than talking with someone who has walked in your shoes. Support groups are available for everything from alcoholism to diabetes to weight control to breast cancer. Start with your local phone book or ask your doctor or therapist for recommendations.

This chapter opened with the story of Al, a victor in his battle against esophageal cancer. Al attributes at least part of his victory to his participation in an Internet support group. Thousands of these groups exist and can be valuable if you're uncomfortable talking with people about your issues in a face-to-face setting.

Whether in person or over the Internet, participating in a support group can lower your anxiety, make you feel less alone, and even help with feelings of depression. But support groups aren't for everyone, and all support groups aren't a positive experience. These tips can help make sure your experience is a good one.

Support Group Support

1. **Find a group that fits.**
   Attending an Alcoholics Anonymous group when you're an occasional drinker who wants to cut back may be overkill. Make sure the group you're attending fits your condition and your circumstances.

2. **Make sure you're comfortable.**
   It's important for you to feel good about the people in the group, how the group is run, and what they're there to accomplish. To make sure you're comfortable with the experience, go to a meeting or two and just observe before you dive in.

3. **Watch for negative influences.**
   It may sound strange, but participating in a support group can sometimes have negative impacts on your condition. Hearing participants' stories may reinforce negative feelings or behaviors, or you may form relationships with people in your group who have a negative rather than a positive impact on your life. For example, support groups for adolescent girls with anorexia have been controversial because the members can actually support dangerous behavior and encourage one another in a negative way. Just monitor your participation to make sure that you're having a positive experience.

4. **Don't give out personal information over the Internet.**
   It's easy to get very comfortable participating in a chat room with other folks who are dealing with the same condition. It may be incomprehensible that someone would pretend they have breast cancer to mislead other people on a site, but it happens every day. Monitor the site without participating to see what course the discussions take. Once you sign on, stay as anonymous as possible until you have participated long enough to know the credibility of the site. If you want to correspond with someone, set up a separate e-mail address from your normal one that you can shut down if the relationship takes a turn you are uncomfortable with. And just keep in mind that anonymous communication always carries the risk of people misrepresenting who they are or their motives.

Your Circle of Positivity

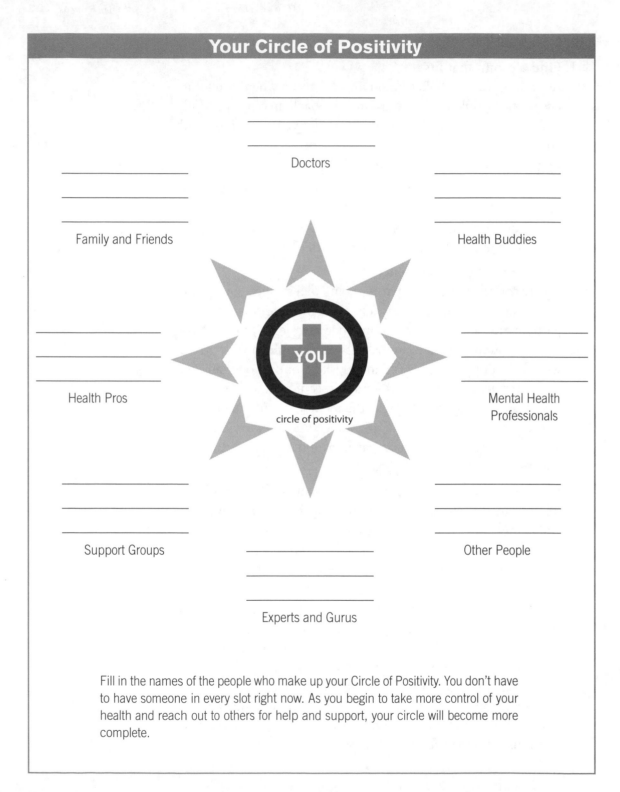

Doctors

Family and Friends

Health Buddies

YOU

circle of positivity

Health Pros

Mental Health Professionals

Support Groups

Other People

Experts and Gurus

Fill in the names of the people who make up your Circle of Positivity. You don't have to have someone in every slot right now. As you begin to take more control of your health and reach out to others for help and support, your circle will become more complete.

5. **Respect the group.**
   Most support groups have rules on confidentiality, trust, and participation. Make sure that you are contributing to the group in a positive way, providing support to other members, and respecting everyone's feelings and privacy.
6. **Know when to leave.**
   It's easy to get attached to the people in your group and to the group experience. Staying in the group as a mentor once you have moved to another level can be a valuable experience, too. But be aware of when your time is up. Staying to hear new

Take the Health Power Challenge

1.	I am ready to fight for my right to be healthy and feel great.	**Yes!**	No
2.	I will not allow fear to keep me from living my healthiest, longest life.	**Yes!**	No
3.	I have a doctor whom I respect, trust, and am honest with.	**Yes!**	No
4.	I am knowledgeable about my health and my vital health information.	**Yes!**	No
5.	I understand that I am responsible for telling my doctor about my conditions, my family history, and what I want from my health.	**Yes!**	No
6.	I am ready to make a commitment to live longer and feel better.	**Yes!**	No
7.	I have the time, energy, and resources to commit to my health.	**Yes!**	No
8.	I understand the effect my choices will have on my health.	**Yes!**	No
9.	I understand how my healthstyle choices impact those I love.	**Yes!**	No
10.	I have the support of my family and friends.	**Yes!**	No
11.	I have a plan for my health to live well with my health conditions.	**Yes!**	No
12.	There is no one who can manage my health better than I can.	**Yes!**	No
13.	I know I may have to face unexpected health challenges.	**Yes!**	No
14.	I am ready to do what it takes to stay healthy and live a long, full life.	**Yes!**	No
15.	**I am ready to take charge of my health, my happiness, and my life!**	**Yes!**	No

members' troubled tales may be too emotionally draining and bring you back to a mental state that you've been able to move on from. Make sure that the group is always a positive influence in your life and that it's helping you move forward, not stagnate.

Are You Ready?

You've cleared out those negative monsters, rejuvenated your Healthy Spirit, and formed your Circle of Positivity. Kick the tires and light the fires—you're ready to go! React to the statements on page 175 honestly and don't worry if you've got a few *no's*. Getting fully powered may take some time. Look at the places where you've still got a *no* and reflect on what you can do to change that to a *yes*!

Your Declaration of Health Independence

In the world we live in today, there aren't many repercussions for ignoring your health. If you don't pay your bills, ignore your taxes, or bounce checks, you can't just pull the covers over your head. You have to face the bill collectors, the IRS, or even the judge.

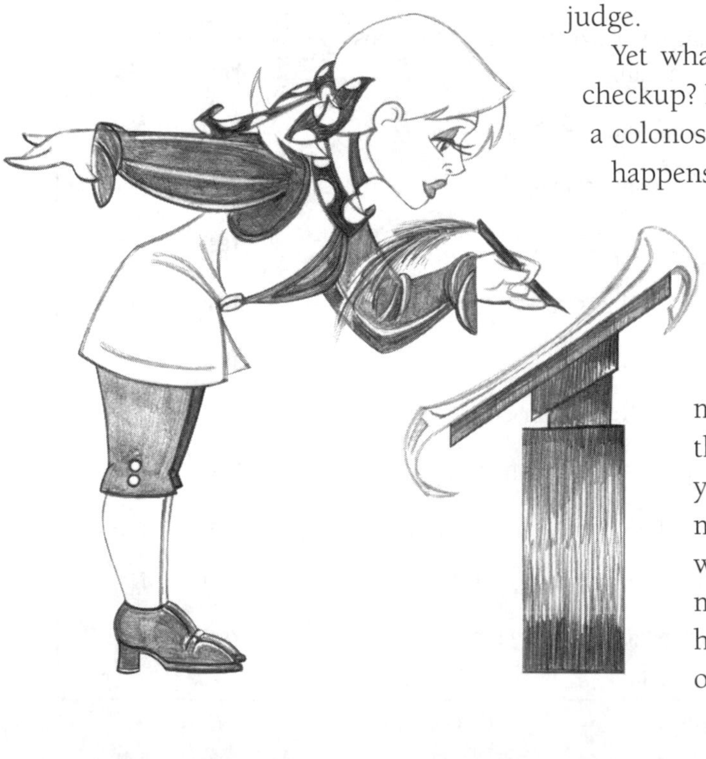

Yet what happens if you don't get an annual checkup? Nothing. What happens if you don't get a colonoscopy when you're fifty? Nothing. What happens if you have diabetes but don't manage your blood sugar? Nothing.

Wait! Wait! Nothing? Not true. You could get a wake-up call a lot worse than one from the IRS. Try the Grim Reaper! I'm exaggerating to make a point, but really, isn't there a little more motivation to have a plan for your health than to have a great retirement plan? Ask anyone, wealthy or not, who's had a serious health challenge how much they would pay to prevent it from happening. The phrase "money is no object" is what usually comes to mind.

Declaration of Health Independence

I hold these truths to be self-evident, that all men and women are created healthy, that they are endowed with certain inalienable privileges, that among these are to live a long life, to feel good, and to be happy. To help secure these privileges, I understand that I am entitled to certain rights from the health care system, the people providing me with care, and those institutions entrusted with promoting, defending, and protecting my health.

Rights

The right to receive care and be treated with respect.
The right to know and approve of who is providing my care.
The right to be given complete, prompt, and accurate information.
The right to refuse treatments I don't want.
The right to expect privacy and confidentiality.
I also understand that in order for me to receive the quality care I am entitled to, I am obliged with certain responsibilities.

Responsibilities

The responsibility to actively participate in my care and decisions about my health.
The responsibility to give accurate, honest information to those giving me care.
The responsibility to agree to and follow treatment plans to the best of my ability.
The responsibility to get regular screenings and to manage my health and conditions.
The responsibility to use health services in a responsible way that respects those giving me care and others seeking care.

I therefore declare that I am a free and independent health consumer, that I am absolved from allegiance to any person or institution not committed to the quality of my health.

In support of this declaration and my Healthy Life Plan, I pledge my Life, my Fortune, and my Sacred Honor.

signed this ____________ *day of* ______________, *the year* ________

by ____

You've done the work it takes to get on track to live longer and feel better. You've faced your fears about your health, looked at your Health Character, gathered knowledge and information about yourself and your health, and developed a Healthy Life Plan. It's time to declare your health independence and make the commitment to take charge of your health and live the long, healthy life you deserve.

Taylor's Seventh Law of Health

Good health is your most important legacy; pass it on.

Prescription 6

Protect Your Family's Health

The Sandwich Generation

"I can't be here," Sarah told the ER nurse as she handed her the gown and told her to get undressed. "I have to go with my mother to her cardiologist appointment and then pick the kids up and take them to the dentist. I can't be here."

"Look," the nurse said. "I can't keep you here and I'm not telling you what to do, but you're having chest pains and that's nothing to fool around with. Did you say your mom has heart problems?"

"Yeah," Sarah responded.

The ER nurse went on, "Well, your doctor obviously took it seriously enough to send you over here. If you'd like me to call your mother or your kids' school, I'd be glad to, but you're not going to be of much use to them if you don't take care of yourself."

Sarah sighed, closed her eyes, lay back, and asked, "How did I wind up here?"

"The hospital?" the nurse asked.

"No," Sarah said, "the kids, the mom, the job, the life!"

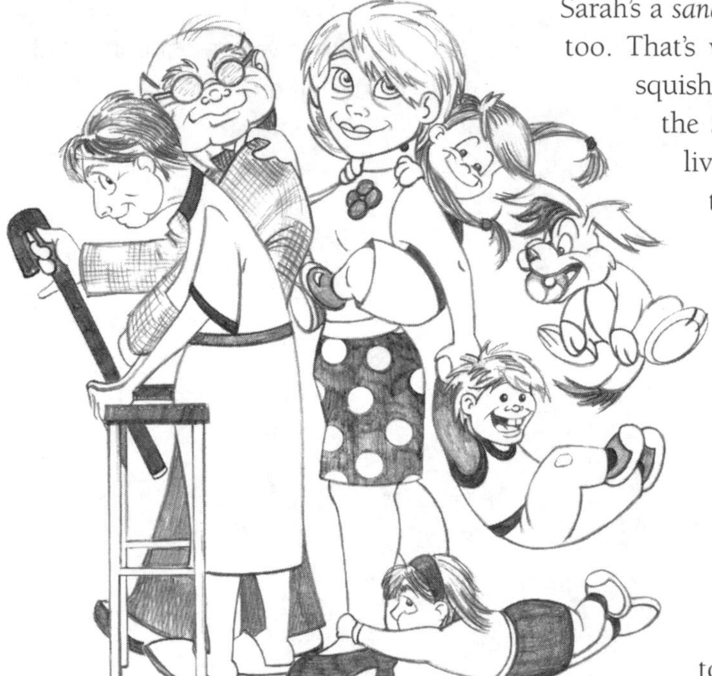

Sarah's a *sandwich*. Chances are you're a sandwich, too. That's what everyone is calling those of us squished between our kids and our parents—the Sandwich Generation. With everyone living longer and people waiting until they're older to have children, the trend is inevitable. When women had kids at twenty and their own parents lived only until about age sixty, these worlds didn't usually collide. Now they're hurtling toward each other on a crash course, and we're all in the middle.

Sarah is a classic sandwich. Stuck between two slices of responsibility, slathered with guilt, and topped off with a nice slice of frustration. Trying to manage everyone's health but neglecting her own. And it's not just women who are squeezed. Our traditional families have morphed into new configurations—single dads, extended families, breadwinner moms, grandparents caring for children while parents work, to name just a few. Men who have their children on the weekends are faced with understanding doctor's appointments and administering allergy medication, and when Grandma moves in, there may not be a wife at home to care for her during the day. Grandparents helping out with the kids have to know what the kids should eat and make sure they get enough exercise and activity.

> There's a thread that binds all of us together. Pull one end, the strain is felt all down the line.
>
> —ROSAMOND MARSHALL, AUTHOR

The upside is that activities such as helping parents manage their medications can help you see things you can do to protect your own health. We're all in this together. We're all living longer, and it's inevitable that each of us will spend a portion of our lives giving care to another family member or loved one. It's estimated that 80 to 98 percent of all in-home long-term care is provided by family members.

You are the center of your family's health—the meat in the sandwich, so to speak. And just like having a plan for your own health, it's critical to your family's well-being that you make healthy habits, safety, and preventive care an important part of your family's life.

Your Family's Health Legacy

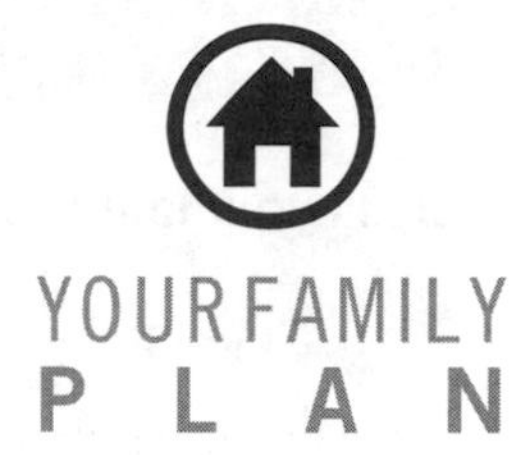

When you think about your family's health legacy, you probably consider an aunt's cancer, your grandfather's diabetes, or your cousin's epilepsy. But a family's health legacy is much broader than that. Although what you inherit genetically is important, what may be more important is the healthstyle habits that are passed down from generation to generation. For example, children of smokers have a much greater chance of becoming smokers themselves. Likewise, if your parents had weight issues, you're at a higher risk for battling the pounds as well. But besides these obvious habits, your health legacy is passed along in thousands of more subtle ways: diet, physical activity, safety, emotional health, positive health images, the importance you place on preventive health.

What's most important is that a family's healthy legacy is not set in stone. From its youngest members to the elders of the tribe, making positive changes to your health will be good for everyone. And the great news is that while inherited physical conditions mean you have to take your risks more seriously, you should know that most inherited conditions, including heart disease, type 2 diabetes, and most cancers, are influenced far more by healthstyle choices than by genes.

The Family Health Inventory beginning on page 182 is a great start to evaluating your family's health and health habits so that your legacy can be one of great health, good humor, and long lives.

With luck, your family has everything together when it comes to your health. But don't feel guilty if there are places that need work. In our busy lives, it's easy to push aside some of the things that are most important—our family's health, safety, and well-being. You're not the only family that eats fast food four nights a week. You're not the only family whose primary form of exercise is getting off the couch to find the remote control.

7 Ways to Get Kids to Take Medicine

Not Just a Spoonful of Sugar

1. *Give medicine only when it's necessary.* This will teach them to use medication only when they need it.
2. *Explain why they have to take it,* how it will make them feel better, and how they will feel if they don't.
3. *Let them be in charge.* Ask them to pick out a spoon or decide where they want to take the medicine. After checking the label (or asking your doctor), let them pick what to drink after taking the medicine.
4. *Make it taste better.* Ask your doctor if you can dip the spoon in chocolate syrup first. This will mask the taste of the medicine.
5. *Don't get into a physical struggle.* It sets up a bad pattern.
6. *Give them an out.* Instead of issuing a punishment, let them choose to walk away and come back when they're calm and ready.
7. *Teach them to swallow pills when they reach school age.* It will make things easier on everyone.

Family Health Inventory

Does your family practice good healthstyle habits?

Circle true or false for each statement.

1.	My family eats a majority of our daily meals together at the dinner table.	**True**	**False**
2.	I do not allow anyone to smoke or use any tobacco products in my house.	**True**	**False**
3.	If anyone in my family consumes alcohol, they do it in moderation and do not drive or operate machinery after drinking.	**True**	**False**
4.	While in the car, my family uses seat belts or age-appropriate car seats at all times.	**True**	**False**
5.	In my house, sedentary activities like watching TV, surfing the Net, and playing video games are kept to a minimum and are time-limited.	**True**	**False**
6.	My family understands the basics of good nutrition and knows approximately how many calories per day they should consume.	**True**	**False**
7.	In my family, we avoid fad diets and focus on good eating habits.	**True**	**False**
8.	In our house, we keep at least one medical reference book to help evaluate the seriousness of symptoms.	**True**	**False**
9.	If an emergency arises where my family cannot make it back to our house (such as a hurricane, an earthquake, a fire, or flooding), we have an established meeting place and a contact person outside our area to inform of our safety.	**True**	**False**
10.	If any member of my family were to need long-term care, we have an established plan that will not financially impact the family and will make sure he or she gets the proper care.	**True**	**False**

Scoring and Evaluation

Evaluation **True** ________ **False** ________

More true than false	You and your family are focused on your health. Great! Keep up the good work and remember that your family is one of the greatest resources for physical and mental health.
Same number true as false	You and your family are on your way to good health. There is no "I" in *team*, but there is in *family*. Take responsibility to keep your family healthy.
More false than true	It's time for a family meeting to discuss all of your health needs and goals. Don't wait until there is a major medical issue to start working together.

Family Health Inventory

Check the pulse of your family's health.

Circle true or false for each statement.

1. We plan active family time together (such as walking, riding bikes, swimming, and gardening).	**True**	**False**
2. We mostly eat a healthy diet of fruits, vegetables, grains, and lean meats, while limiting processed foods that are high in sugar and fat.	**True**	**False**
3. We have a written record of our family health history to help us determine if there are any predispositions to diseases.	**True**	**False**
4. Everyone in our family knows how to dial 9-1-1, where the first aid kit is, what the symptoms of a heart attack are, and how to administer CPR.	**True**	**False**
5. Every member of the family gets an annual health exam and age-appropriate screenings.	**True**	**False**
6. My family is covered by a health insurance plan so we do not have to worry about the cost of basic medical treatment.	**True**	**False**
7. We all have written advance directives that we have talked about with our family members.	**True**	**False**
8. Everyone in the family is up to date on their immunizations as well as any necessary tests or screenings.	**True**	**False**
9. We talk regularly about what health is, how we can stay healthy, and what good health means to our family.	**True**	**False**
10. Everyone in the family has a primary care physician we trust for regular checkups and to help us with our larger medical decisions.	**True**	**False**

Scoring and Evaluation

Evaluation	**True** ________ **False** ________
More true than false	Your family has a good plan for your health. Make sure you stick with your plan to emphasize prevention, healthy habits, and family support.
Same number true as false	Your family members are aware of their health, but may need a little encouragement from you to get everything up to date.
More false than true	You've got some work to do. You may be neglecting important steps to keep your family members healthy and well. First, get everyone up to date on checkups and screenings and make sure you're prepared for emergencies.

(continued)

Family Health Inventory (continued)

How well do you work together as a family?

Circle true or false for each statement.

1.	In our family, we focus on each person's strengths and not on their size or appearance.	**True**	**False**
2.	We encourage one another to develop and practice talents and special interests that we each possess.	**True**	**False**
3.	Even with our hectic schedules, we make time for recreation, rest, relaxation, and fun.	**True**	**False**
4.	If a member of our family is going through a stressful time, we support him and help him through his stressful period.	**True**	**False**
5.	When a family member becomes angry, we try to identify the source of the anger and work toward a resolution before a crisis occurs.	**True**	**False**
6.	We don't overschedule our time or allow one person's needs to dominate all of our family time. We allow everyone to feel that their needs are just as important.	**True**	**False**
7.	We have established family ground rules. That way everyone knows which behaviors are acceptable and which are not.	**True**	**False**
8.	We can talk about important issues facing the family without getting angry at one another.	**True**	**False**
9.	Our family members are the most important people to us; we will not allow outside influences to come between us.	**True**	**False**
10.	We are not afraid to get outside help for issues like substance abuse, mental issues, anger management, or family conflicts.	**True**	**False**

Scoring and Evaluation

Evaluation **True** _________ **False** _________

More true than false	You work well together to support one another emotionally. Make sure you stay on top of any issues and resolve them quickly.
Same number true as false	You have a close family unit, but may not always be sensitive to one another's needs. It's time to take inventory and see where you can do better!
More false than true	Your family may benefit from some outside perspective. Some members may have issues they're not comfortable talking about, and a little help on communication and conflict resolution could set you on the right track.

At the end of the day, when you all come trudging home after work, after school, after soccer, after whatever, facing three hours of homework, a pile of dirty laundry, and everyone tired and hungry, it's only natural to look for the easy way out. But what may seem easy at the time can cost you in terms of your family's mental and physical well-being.

And the same goes for preventive health. As parents and children, we all know it's important that everyone from baby to Great-grandma get annual checkups, watch the medicine they take, and get the screenings and exams they need. But what you might not be aware of is how important it is to be your family's health advocate. Medical mistakes and lack of care have the greatest effect on the most vulnerable—our children and our senior adults. A harmless dose of the wrong medication in a healthy adult may be fatal if given to a child. Likewise, while you might simply go to bed for a few days to battle the flu, a bout with the flu for your mom or dad could have devastating effects on their health, including pneumonia, respiratory

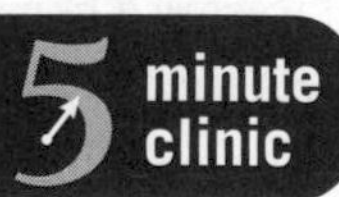

6 Habits of Healthy Families

1. **They eat together.** Experts say the more meals you eat at home, the healthier everyone eats. It's a great bonding experience and will cut both calories and costs. Also, don't just stand at a kitchen counter, sit down together at the table.
2. **They play together.** A family that is active together is closer *and* healthier. Families that schedule activities together do a much better job of sticking with it and staying healthy.
3. **They have healthy routines.** Brushing their teeth, reasonable bedtimes, wearing seat belts, healthy snacking—these types of good routines help keep everyone in the family on track and feeling great.
4. **They talk openly about health.** They talk to their kids about school, about drugs, about sex. Don't neglect the most important part of their maturity—their health. They talk about what it means to be healthy, what you give up when you're not, and how you can be healthy throughout your life.
5. **They emphasize prevention.** They have annual checkups, a major part of protecting lives and health. They make sure everyone has a primary care doctor, sees her at least once a year, and gets whatever screenings they need. They also keep a family health history and have organized records about everyone's vital health info.
6. **They have a happy home.** Supporting one another through thick and thin is key to having a healthy family. Also, it's important to have balance so that no one dominates the family, either with activities, stress, problems, friends, or anything else. Be there for one another and be willing to ask for help from others when you need it.

conditions, and worse. Seventy thousand Americans over sixty-five die unnecessarily every year from illnesses that can be prevented or mitigated by two-dollar shots.

In this chapter we're going to take a look at four different aspects of your family's health: Protecting Children, Issues for Women, Health for Men, and Healthy Aging. I'll tell you how to protect your kids from medical mistakes, how to keep your mind sharp as you get older, and how to know when someone needs help. I'll also address special health concerns for women, and the one thing that will finally get men to take better care of their health.

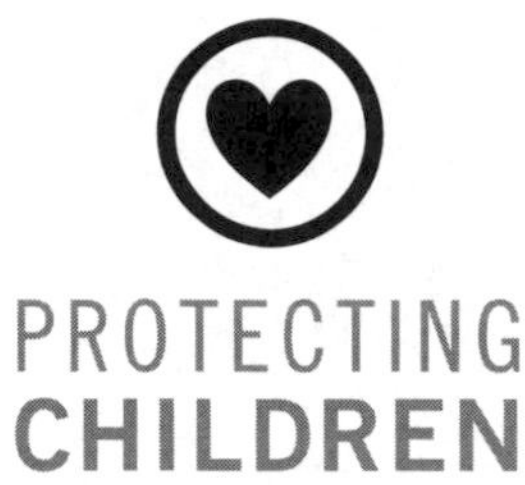

Protecting Children from Medical Mistakes

When it comes to your children, grandchildren, nephews, nieces, or the children of friends, take everything you've learned in this book about taking charge of your health and multiply it by ten. If it's important for you to have knowledge about your health, reclaim your health power, and make sure you choose the right doctors for yourself, children need all of this and more. A study out of Harvard Medical School shows that medical errors with the potential to cause harm occur in children's care three times more often than in adult care. And children can't handle these medical mistakes as well as adults, physically or emotionally. Children's bodies are more delicate. Their bodies—their nervous system, their heart, their lungs, their brain, and their bones—are all still developing and are more vulnerable. A medical mistake that might be easily tolerated by an adult could have devastating effects on a child's development, causing her lifelong problems.

That's why children need a health advocate to monitor and manage their care at all times. They are too young to question what is happening. They can't speak for themselves and don't have the experience or knowledge to know if they are getting a medication, a treatment, or a diagnosis that could be dangerous to them. They may also have difficulty understanding and communicating side effects or symptoms. Doctors will tell you that their most important source of information about a patient's status is often the patient himself. Lab reports and tests can't tell them everything, so doctors rely on patients to describe their symptoms, tell them how much pain they're in, and let the doctor know if they're feeling better or worse. When young patients have difficulty communicating this information, having a parent who knows them well and can interpret their behaviors and descriptions is critical.

A Devastating Loss and Unnecessary Pain

Even when parents are deeply involved and have the best medical care at their disposal, mistakes and lack of communication can have devastating results. Sorrel King, an advocate for improving patient safety, speaks from personal experience. Her daughter Josie died in the hospital at Johns Hopkins Children's Center while being treated for burns from a bathtub accident—not from her primary injuries, but, as the hospital admitted, from a total breakdown in the system. A series of miscommunications and a lack of coordination resulted in the eighteen-month-old girl suffering catastrophic brain damage after her heart stopped because of severe dehydration. The medical staff hadn't responded appropriately to the obvious warning signs—dramatic weight loss, severe diarrhea, intense thirst, and lethargy. To

Ask, Know, Go

Protect Your Child's Life in the Hospital

Children who are in the hospital for any reason are at particular risk. Hospitals are primarily designed to deal with the health issues of "big people," including most of their equipment and staff. An assumption is made that patients can speak for themselves, which children most often cannot. If your child is in the hospital, you or another family member or friend should be with her at all times to make sure she is safe and taken care of. Use this tactic to keep her safe:

When someone is doing a test or a procedure on your child or giving her a medication

ASK what they are doing and why.

KNOW exactly what will happen and understand risks.

GO with your child to make sure she is comfortable and no mistakes are made.

Do not allow yourself to feel as if you are being overbearing, and don't be intimidated into leaving your child alone. She is your child, and it is your job to keep her safe. As well intentioned as every doctor, nurse, or technician is, it is you and your child who will have to live with any mistakes or negative outcomes.

5 minute clinic: 6 Medical Mistakes That Affect Kids and How to Avoid Them

Mistakes affect children more seriously than adults. Protect your child from these errors.

1. **Medication.** This is by far the most common medical mistake in children. Be sure they are taking the correct medication, in the right amount for their weight and at the right time. Double-check with the doctor and the pharmacist that everything is correct before giving any drugs to your child.
2. **In the hospital.** Most medical mistakes happen in the hospital. If your child is hospitalized, someone needs to be with him as his advocate *at all times*. Children often can't describe a symptom or understand the directions they are given. *Never* leave them alone.
3. **Allergies.** Tell your doctor and pharmacist about any known or possible allergies or adverse reactions your child may have had to medications, food, or other substances.
4. **Surgical errors.** Children have special surgical needs. If you have a choice, choose a doctor and a facility where many of the same pediatric procedures have been performed. Experience is essential for a good outcome.
5. **Emergency room (1).** Do not use the ER for your child's routine medical treatment. The ER doctors do not know your child's medical history, possibly leading to medical mistakes. Your child must have a primary care doctor.
6. **Emergency room (2).** Before an emergency arises, make sure you know which facility in your area is equipped to handle the needs of a child. In a major emergency always call 9-1-1. The EMTs are experts in knowing which facilities can handle your needs.

hear stories of the child trying to communicate her condition—sucking on a washcloth while being bathed, screaming "mo, mo!" when given a drink—brings tears to your eyes. Richard Kidwell, Johns Hopkins managing attorney on the case, said that the hospital staff should have listened more closely to the girl's mother, who had repeatedly expressed worries about her daughter's decline. "Nobody knows a child better than the parents," he said. Today, Johns Hopkins and Sorrel King are working together to try to change a flawed system that causes untold pain to thousands of families every day.

This example is extreme, but mistakes happen constantly in our health care system, and when the mistake involves a child, it is that much more devastating. A study of medication errors involving children found that in a review of 10,000 orders, 600 contained medication errors. One contributing factor is that almost all drug doses for children have to be calculated. Very few drugs exist in dosages for children, so doctors and nurses have to calculate the percentage of an adult dose based on the body weight of the child. Pharmacists often dilute stock solutions or divide pills—an imprecise procedure that opens the door for mistakes.

No one—no doctor, nurse, pharmacist, or technician—is infallible. And yet our health care system is organized around just that assumption. When you examine the system, you'll see there are few checks and balances. Everyone assumes that what the person in front of them did is correct. That's why simple mistakes can keep compounding until they reach lethal proportions. When a child is involved, that final check and balance—patient approval—is often missing. Nothing is more stressful than when your child is hurt or sick—you'll do and say anything just to make them better. Of course you're grateful to the dedicated nurses, technicians, and physicians who are caring for your child. But your role in his care is the most important of all. You are there to speak for him when he can't, to protect him when no one else can, and to keep tabs on a system that often doesn't keep tabs on itself. There are things every parent and caregiver should know about their child's health that could save his life.

8 Things Parents Must Know about Their Child's Health

1. **What is being done to your child and why**
   When someone is doing a test or a procedure on your child, providing her with medical care, or giving her a medication, don't be shy. Ask every person who works on your child what they are doing and why they are doing it. Approach every transaction as an opportunity to correct a mistake. I know it sounds harsh, but your child's life may be at stake. Use the ASK, KNOW, GO tactic to make sure your child is always protected.
2. **Your child's weight in kilograms**
   Drug doses for children are usually calculated by the child's weight in kilograms. Know your child's weight and confirm it with any doctor or nurse who is prescribing or administering a medication. Here's how you can convert your child's weight:

   Child's weight in pounds _________ divided by
   2.2 = _________ weight in kilograms.
3. **Your child's health history, conditions, and allergies**
   A written list is the way to go. Allergies are more common and can be more dangerous in children. If your child has a life-threatening allergy, make sure she wears a Medic Alert bracelet. Include any other important information on your child's health history or medical conditions.
4. **Every medication your child takes**
   Keep a written list and give it to anyone caring for your child (doctor, nurse, hospital staff). A drug interaction can be deadly for a child. Include vitamins, over-the-counter drugs, and supplements.

5. **Five critical questions about every medication**
   Anytime your child is given a prescription or administered a medication (especially in a hospital), ask these five critical questions.
   1. What are you giving him?
   2. What is it for?
   3. What is the dosage, and how was it calculated?
   4. How is it given? (Make sure you understand how to do it.)
   5. What are the side effects or adverse effects?

   Don't be embarrassed or feel you are being annoying—*You are your child's only advocate!* Confirm this information every step of the way—with the doctors, with the nurses, with the pharmacist. Something as small as a misplaced decimal point can result in a child's death. Mistakes are made every day—assume the worst and you'll get the best.

6. **How your child feels**
   When your child is ill, and you are at the doctor's office or the hospital, pay close attention to how she feels and to any changes in her condition. A child's medical condition can deteriorate rapidly, so stayed tuned in to how she's feeling and demand attention immediately if you are worried.

7. **Who's watching out for your child**
   If your child is in the hospital with an acute condition, you or another adult you trust should be with your child around the clock to oversee his care. If *you* think doctors and nurses are intimidating, imagine your child's fears. Children are taught to listen to and respect adults, so it's very difficult for them to question someone giving them care.

8. **Your doctor's experience treating children**
   Pediatric medicine is not "adult medicine only smaller." Children's organs and systems are more delicate and react differently than adults. Children respond differently to emergencies and describe symptoms differently (for example, children who are nauseated typically say their "tummy hurts.") Make sure that the doctors who are treating your child are experienced with children.

For the Record

Ask any parent to see a picture of their kids and *whoosh!* out comes the wallet or photo album faster than you can say, "Is that Play-Doh on your carpet?" But ask those same parents to show you their children's health records and you'll most likely get a blank stare and a "What?" Hey, I'm not throwing stones. From a bead shoved up my son Jack's nose to my daughter Sam's close encounter in the face with a piñata stick (ouch!), I've arrived at plenty of emergency room visits armed with nothing more than a scared kid and a teary-eyed mom (me). Not to mention the blank look on my face when my children's pediatrician would ask if they were up to date on their shots and when their last checkup had been. This isn't a matter of caring about your child or being irresponsible.

RESOURCE

Keep Your Kids' Health Information Handy

Order a Kid's Essential Health Organizer at www.tayloryourhealth.com.

Your Child's Must-Have Health Documents

Authorization for Emergency Treatment

This form grants permission for someone other than you to authorize emergency medical treatment for your child—for example, babysitters, school officials, grandparents. Without a signed consent form, a hospital may wait until they can reach you to provide medical care to your child. You can find a free form to download for your use at www.tayloryourhealth.com.

Written Health History

Vital information about your child's health should include:

- medications and allergies
- a history of health conditions, hospital stays, tests, and treatments
- a checkup schedule and records
- an immunization schedule
- a family health history (include grandparents, sisters and brothers, aunts and uncles)

List of Emergency Contacts

Keep a list of people to contact in case of an emergency. Include doctors, teachers, relatives, caregivers, neighbors, friends, and family. Give your child a copy of the list and talk about when she might need to contact someone for help (for example, if you are sick or injured, in case of a natural disaster, or if she is lost or separated from you). Talking calmly to children about situations that might arise and how they should handle them can give them a sense of power over their own safety and will help them be prepared for situations.

Talking to Kids about Health

1. If your child's not feeling well or has a medical condition, offer him a little extra TLC. It's okay to baby him right now.
2. Encourage them to talk about their health fears, including death.
3. Answer their questions as honestly as you can in a way that's appropriate to their age.
4. If your child is getting treatment or going to the doctor, talk honestly about what will happen. Surprises aren't fun for anyone. But don't give him so much detail that it upsets him.
5. Keep a positive outlook yourself.

The norm in our society is to walk around in a stupor about our children's health (as we often do about our own), relying on someone else to keep the records, someone else to remind us of checkups, someone else to help them if there's an emergency. But it's time for everyone to face reality—parents, grandparents, caregivers, that someone else is you! You are the sole keeper of your children's records and health history. You hold the key to giving your children and their doctors vital information that will help keep them healthy now and when they become adults.

Giving your children a complete health history that includes their family health tree can be one of the most important gifts you will ever give. Each of us inherits a unique set of risks from our mothers, fathers, grandparents, and other ancestors. The sooner your children can identify those risks, the sooner they and their doctors can develop a plan to make sure they practice healthy habits and combat any hereditary risks they face with early testing, diagnosis, and treatment. Very few conditions are inevitable if addressed early enough with the right plan.

Surprising Health Problems for Kids

Backpacks

Overloaded backpacks are putting kids at risk for serious shoulder and back pain—92 percent of kids worldwide frequently complain of pain.

Lunch boxes

An environmental group found that soft-vinyl lunch boxes contain lead, either in the lining or the exterior plastic, possibly exposing children to what could become an unhealthy level.

Fluoride

Dentists warn that cavities are making a comeback, due to the excessive use of bottled water, most of which doesn't contain the fluoride added to tap water decades ago to reduce tooth decay.

Prescription drugs

A growing drug-abuse threat to teens and youngsters is coming from a new source—the family medicine cabinet. According to an annual study on teen drug abuse, for the first time teens are more likely to have experimented with prescription drugs such as Vicodin and Oxycontin rather than illegal drugs like marijuana. And one in eleven teens said they had abused over-the-counter drugs such as cough medicine or cold tablets, causing one researcher to label today's kids "Generation Rx."

A mom from New York City, who had been given one of my Kid's Pocket Health Organizers for her child, filled out his important info and placed it in his backpack (he managed asthma). She called me after the 2003 blackout to tell me how relieved she was that she had given her son information on when to take his medication and what to do if he couldn't reach her in an emergency. She was still worried, but remarked on how such a small thing had given her peace of mind. The time to give your child emergency information is not when a crisis strikes, but now, when you can calmly talk about what to do.

6 Health Habits Every Parent Should Teach Their Kids

1. Wash their hands.
2. Brush their teeth twice a day.
3. Choose healthy foods.
4. Be safe.
5. Be physically active.
6. Have fun and be happy.

As your child grows, include her in building and maintaining her own health information. Not only will she have the information when she needs it, you will have helped create a heightened sense of responsibility for her health and helped her understand and embrace things she can do to be healthier as a child and as an adult. Most importantly, she will grow up understanding that she is her own best health advocate.

Myths about a Woman's Heart

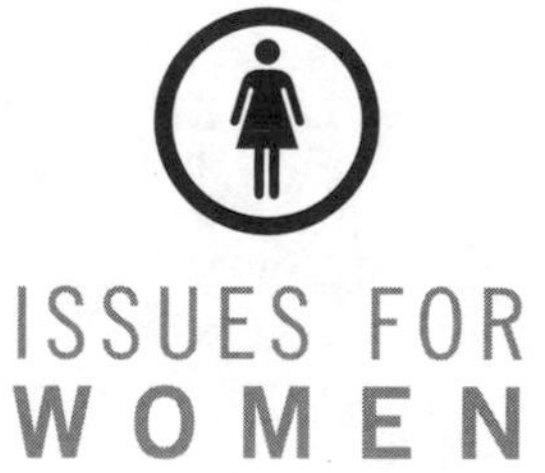

Heart disease is a serious condition affecting millions of women around the globe. The troubling news is that most women say that it's not a subject their doctor has ever brought up. The good news is that there are a lot of things you can do to reduce your risk of getting heart disease, make your heart healthier, and get treatment in time to save your life if you do have a heart problem or attack. Let's take a look at some of the myths surrounding heart disease and women and what every woman can do to protect her heart and her life.

Heart Myth: Breast cancer is the leading cause of death in women.

Heart Facts

- Around 40,000 women each year die from breast cancer.
- Heart disease kills over 350,000 women each year.
- Heart disease kills more women than the next sixteen leading causes of death combined.
- A woman has a 4 percent chance of dying from breast cancer and a 33 percent chance of dying from heart disease.

Could It Be a Heart Attack?

Know the Symptoms

- Chest pains or tightness in chest (If you are over seventy-five, have diabetes, or have had a previous heart attack, you may not experience chest pains.)
- Pain radiating down arms, particularly the left arm
- Indigestion, nausea, or vomiting
- Heart palpitations (your heart beating rapidly)
- Weakness or dizziness
- Shortness of breath
- Anxiety or a sense of impending doom or dread

Get Treatment Fast—Minutes Can Save Your Life

- Call 9-1-1 or go to the Emergency Room.
- Chew an aspirin (real aspirin, not Tylenol, Motrin, or Advil).
- If your doctor gave you nitroglycerin tablets, use them according to your doctor's instructions. Do not take nitroglycerin unless you have been given it by your doctor.
- If your heart stops, the closest person should call 9-1-1; then someone who is trained should begin CPR or use a defibrillator to restart the heart.

Get Medical Assistance Immediately.

Heart Myth: Heart disease is a man's problem.

Heart Facts

- Women are more likely than men to have a silent heart attack, which can be undetectable while damaging your heart.
- Most research on treating heart disease has been conducted on men, even though men's and women's hearts react differently.
- Women who are in the hospital for heart problems are twice as likely to die as men.

Heart Myth: Heart disease affects only women who are overweight.

Heart Facts

- It's estimated that one in four women in America have some type of heart disease.

- Even women at a healthy weight can have high cholesterol or blood pressure and can suffer "silent" heart attacks that damage their hearts.

Heart Myth: Having heart disease means you will have a heart attack.

Heart Facts

- Heart disease comes in many forms, including atherosclerosis (blocked arteries to the heart), stroke, arrhythmia, and congestive heart failure.
- Heart disease does not always result in a heart attack. By making changes to your healthstyle habits, you can often combat the effects of heart disease and have a long, full life.

Heart Myth: Most smokers die from lung cancer.

Heart Facts

- While lung cancer is, of course, a major cause for concern if you smoke, smoking actually kills more people through heart disease than through lung cancer.

Heart Myth: Most people who have a heart attack die.

Heart Facts

- Two-thirds of people who have heart attacks survive.
- Doctors estimate that 375,000 people die each year from heart attacks who might have been saved if they had received quick treatment.
- Chewing an aspirin (real aspirin, not Tylenol, Motrin, or Advil) right away if you are experiencing heart attack symptoms can save your life.

The most important thing to know about your heart health is that it's primarily in your hands. The top nine risk factors for heart attacks are all things that are within your control. I'm not saying they're all easy, but at least you can develop a plan to attack them (no pun intended) one by one to have the healthiest heart you can. Even if you inherited a condition or were born with a heart defect (about 300,000 women in the United States have a congenital heart condition), making changes to your healthstyle is the best way to keep it ticking loud and strong.

Top 9 Heart Risks

1. Weight
2. Lack of physical activity
3. Smoking
4. Unhealthy diet
5. Alcohol
6. High blood pressure
7. High cholesterol
8. Diabetes
9. Mental health (stress, depression)

5 minute clinic

8 Heart Don'ts That Might Surprise You

1. **Don't diet.** Diets don't work. Instead, the key is to change your eating habits. Writing down everything you eat will help you decrease your calories.
2. **Don't exercise.** What!? The key to getting consistent exercise is to find physical activities you can do and make them a part of your everyday routine.
3. **Don't worry about stress.** Worrying about your stress is just too stressful! Try to avoid things that give you anxiety and learn to take more of life in stride.
4. **Don't give up alcohol.** If you don't drink, you may not want to start, but several studies have shown that one or two glasses of red wine a day can help lower your heart disease risk.
5. **Don't smoke.** If you smoke, make it your number-one priority to quit—period. It is the best move, by far, you can make for your health.
6. **Don't ignore the warnings.** Learn the warning signs of a heart attack and get *immediate* medical assistance. But you'll also need to pay attention to the more subtle signs of heart disease: elevated blood pressure, high cholesterol, unhealthy weight, diabetes.
7. **Don't do it yourself.** Find a great doctor whom you trust to assess your heart health, check your vital signs, and get you on a treatment plan if you need it.
8. **Don't hope for the best.** Don't just sit back with your fingers crossed, hoping you won't get heart disease. Get informed about your health and your heart, work with your doctor to figure out your risks, and take control of your health to get the tests, prevention, and treatment you need.

Guilt by Association

From spending too much money to not paying enough attention to the kids to sneaking cupcakes on your diet, American women have a knack for piling on the guilt. Guilt is defined as not being able to forgive yourself for a perceived wrongdoing. When it's healthy, guilt can make you correct negative actions and apologize to those you might have hurt. The key is being able to distinguish between a real wrongdoing, where you need to take responsibility for your actions, and something you believe you did wrong that might not have harmed anyone, yet you can't let it go.

Not surprisingly, psychologists say that women handle guilt very differently than men do. Most men feel guilt (yes, girls, they really do), but they don't seem to dwell on it as much, while women seem to beat themselves up a lot more.

But what's so bad about carrying a little unresolved guilt? The problem isn't the guilt. The trouble comes when it eats away at your self-esteem, keeping you from moving forward or focusing too much on what others think of you. Unresolved guilt over an issue that goes on for a long time or guilt that resurfaces with everything you do can lead to other mental conditions like anxiety and even depression.

Everyone feels guilt, but some are more prone to guilty feelings than others. Some qualities that may make you vulnerable to excessive guilt include:

- a need for control
- an obsession with being perfect
- low self-esteem
- holding onto issues and anger

If your guilt is about an event that you have hung onto for years or if it is turning into depression or overwhelming you, consider getting professional help from a mental health therapist. A therapist can

How to Let Go of Your Guilt

The best way to resolve your feelings of guilt is to replace them with feelings of responsibility. By acknowledging what your responsibility is in a situation, you can figure out if you have anything to really feel guilty about. If so, you can try to apologize and make amends to anyone who was hurt—if not, you can let it go. Try asking yourself these questions if you find yourself feeling guilty.

What do I feel guilty about? Try to pinpoint the exact situation that is causing these feelings—not making cookies for your son's class, talking harshly to a coworker, buying an outfit you can't afford.

Was anyone hurt by what I did? Truly hurt, not just a hurt that you're imagining. If you aren't sure, work up the courage to ask. You may be surprised at how many times you are exaggerating a hurt that isn't there. If not, the person you hurt may feel better just because you asked.

If I hurt someone, can I make it up to them? Usually the simplest solution is to just apologize.

What can I do to change my behavior so the situation doesn't occur again? If you found yourself snapping at your husband for leaving his dirty socks on the floor, try talking to him about how helpful it would be if everyone could pick up after themselves. Or realize that in the big picture of life, socks on the floor maybe isn't so bad.

Is it time to let go of my guilt? If you've answered all the questions above and taken positive action, the answer is no doubt *yes*!

5 minute clinic — 11 Risk Factors for Osteoporosis

Risk Factors You Can't Change

- **Being a woman.** Although men can suffer bone fractures, too, women start out with smaller, less-dense bones than men, raising their risk.
- **Getting older.** As we all get older, it's just a fact that our bones get thinner.
- **Having a small frame.** Being especially thin may put you at a greater risk for bone loss as you age. But heavier people get it, too.
- **Family history.** A family history of fractures or osteoporosis may mean you have a higher risk.
- **Going through menopause.** After menopause, your body produces less estrogen, a hormone that protects your bones.
- **Being Caucasian or Asian.** These groups are at a higher risk, although Hispanic and African American women are not immune.

Risk Factors You Can Change

- **Not getting enough calcium and vitamin D.** Your body needs vitamin D to help it absorb calcium, which is crucial to building strong bones throughout your life.
- **Eating disorders.** Anorexia or bulimia can rob your body of the essential nutrients it needs to build strong bones.
- **Smoking.** Smoking increases loss of bone mass.
- **Inactivity.** The less physically active you are, the more bone loss you will experience as you age.
- **Drinking too much alcohol.** While the link between alcohol and loss of bone density is in question, we do know that women who drink have a higher rate of bone fractures from accidents.

help you identify the source of your guilt and work through it so you can move on to a positive place.

Bad to the Bone

Osteoporosis is a condition that robs your bones of their strength by making them less dense, more brittle, and more prone to break. It affects 50 percent of women over the age of forty-five and 90 percent of women over seventy-five, causing over 25,000 hip fractures every year. Throughout your life your bones reform as you lose old bone and replace it with new tissue. As you grow older, more bone is broken down than is replaced, leaving you with spaces inside your bones that look like spiderwebs. As osteoporosis worsens, the spaces in the spiderweb grow bigger as the threads and outer shell of your bones become thinner.

Like high blood pressure, osteoporosis is a silent disease. You don't usually have any symptoms until you have a broken bone. You may lose partial inches off your height, but it is often too gradual to notice. Measuring your height once a year is an easy way to check the health of your bones.

Although doctors recommend getting a bone density test after age sixty-five to assess if you have any bone loss and how much, you can't wait until then to start protecting your bones. Making sure you get enough calcium in your diet should begin as early as possible in life—during childhood is best. So if you have daughters, make sure you watch their diet to be certain they're building strong bones. The amount of milk your daughter drinks between the ages of nine and eighteen

Got Calcium?

Some sources of calcium are obvious . . .

- Milk (whole, 2 percent, 1 percent, and skim)
- Cheese
- Yogurt
- Fruit juices (like OJ) that have been fortified with calcium

Others, not so much . . .

- Canned fish with bones you can eat (salmon and sardines)
- Dark green veggies like kale, collard greens, and broccoli
- Bread made from calcium-fortified flour
- Margarine and other spreads fortified with calcium
- Tofu
- Legumes (beans, baked beans, peas)
- Seeds and nuts (almonds, sesame seeds)
- Total breakfast cereal (has 100 percent of the daily recommended calcium!)

is a large determinant of how strong her bones will be later in life. Teenage girls need four eight-ounce glasses every day. Skim or 2 percent milk works fine and doesn't add so many extra calories.

If you or your daughters have trouble getting enough calcium in your diet, you can also try chewing several Tums a day. They are packed with calcium and are an inexpensive, tasty alternative to supplements.

Being physically active throughout your life is also another important key to building strong bones. Weight-bearing activities like walking, jogging, and playing tennis are best. While great for your heart and your muscles, stretching activities like yoga or aerobic activities such as swimming won't contribute to building your bones. Exercises that strengthen your back muscles are also important, as they will help support your spine and prevent you from developing a stooped posture as you get older. Ask your doctor to recommend some exercises that will help with your back. If you have a family history of severe osteoporosis, you should also ask your doctor to refer you to a specialist who can help you develop a prevention strategy and also a physical therapist who can assist with an exercise program that will work for you.

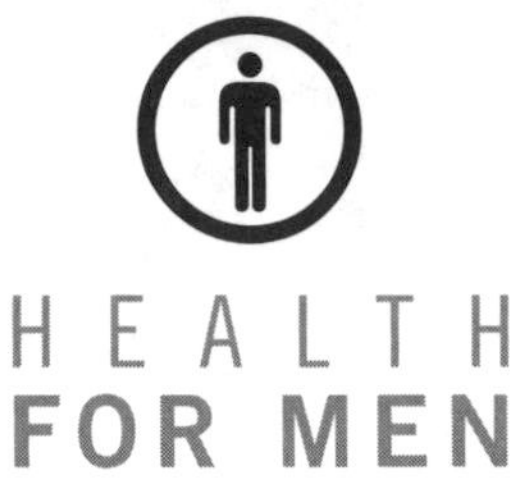

Men—It's All about the Little Guy

What's with men and health anyway? It's not so much that men don't care about their health, but we've all been socialized to believe that somehow it's not "manly" to be too concerned with your health. Dr. Jean Bonhomme, a consultant to the Men's Health Network, views it as an issue that starts early in a man's life. "From the time that boys are young they are taught that it's brave and strong to ignore pain. The result is that men have been taught to minimize and ignore the symptoms of their own bodies." Things that girls take for granted from an early age—annual exams, preventive tests—young men just don't consider a necessary part of how they feel. According to Dr. Bonhomme, the majority of men surveyed said that even if they are sick, they put off seeing a doctor as long as possible. "There's this feeling among men that if they aren't on their deathbed, they're not going to seek medical care."

The 7 Funniest Nicknames for the "Little Guy"

1. The littlest traffic cop
2. Donald Pump
3. President Johnson
4. The Exxon Valdenis
5. Chief of Staff
6. The New York Post
7. Pennis the Menace

That statement may be closer to the truth than most men realize. This lack of concern and care for their health actually puts you on your deathbed, on average, six years sooner than women. Of the fifteen leading causes of death in the United States, men lead women in all fifteen. A doctor once said to me, "You don't want the body of a woman before fifty or the body of a man after fifty." I don't know about that, but I kind of see his point. It seems that women go through a lot of health issues throughout their lives, from periods to pregnancy to menopause. Men, for the most part, just skate on through until *wham!* they get hit by heart disease, prostate issues, diabetes, and so on. But that scenario isn't all that it seems. First, women have their share of health issues as they get older, too, many of them the same as men's. And men's health problems don't just appear out of nowhere—it just seems as if they do. But many of the symptoms are brewing for a lot longer. It's just tough to get you guys to the doctor to do a little preventive maintenance before your engine blows up.

But let's get real. There is one thing that will drive a man to the doctor faster than a Porsche Carrera—problems with the "little guy." You know what I'm talking about.

The biggest mistake you can make is thinking that things like heart disease, diabetes, and cancer won't affect you until you're older and you'll deal with it then. But let's talk turkey. I don't know many (any?) men who would say they plan to stop having sex when they're fifty. But the reality is that if you begin to experience symptoms of heart disease, diabetes, and other chronic conditions, you may not have a choice in the matter. Take a look at the top seven causes of physical impotence.

1. Heart disease
2. Diabetes
3. Nervous system diseases
4. Cancer surgery
5. Medications
6. Substance abuse
7. Hormone imbalance

You'll notice that the vast percentage of these causes are preventable or altogether avoidable simply by adopting good health habits at an early age, getting preventive health services, and having a good plan for your health.

The problem is that if you wait to start worrying about high blood pressure until you're fifty or sixty, by then your options for treatment can be limited and almost certainly will include medication, which will

Top 7 Causes of Impotence

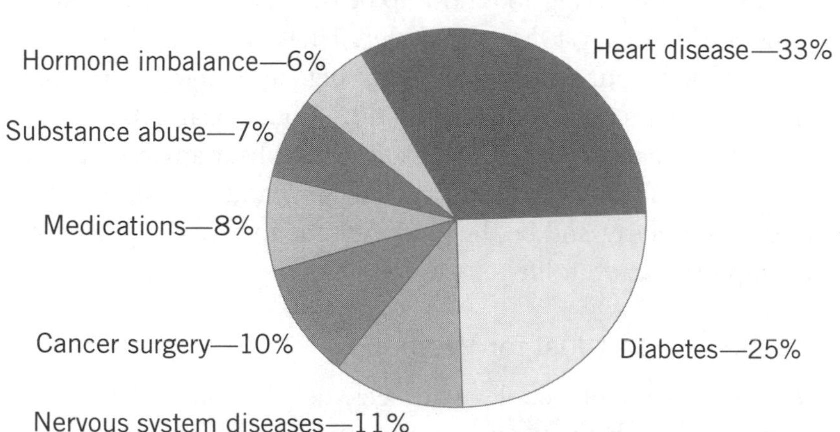

5 minute clinic

7 Reasons Men Don't Like Going to the Doctor

What, me? I'm fine. I don't need to go to the doctor! Now, could you please help me get up?

1. **I'm not a sissy.** Men are taught from an early age that they are weak if they show emotion or express physical discomfort. Going to the doctor can cause both to happen.
2. **Late bloomers.** Men have fewer health issues than women do before the age of forty. Men usually go to the doctor only when something goes wrong. After forty, men will get the opportunity to know their doctor much better.
3. **Don't judge me.** Men think that their situation is unique to them. Don't worry, your doctor has been there and done that.
4. **Satisfaction not guaranteed.** Men find it easy to dismiss things they are not comfortable with by putting them down. Going to the doctor is a "waste of time," "costs too much," and "he doesn't do anything." While sometimes that's true, finding a doctor you are comfortable with can help.
5. **Women and children first.** Most men think that doctors' practices are geared toward women and children. Many men aren't comfortable telling the female receptionist that they are having trouble with their "little guy."
6. **Work comes first.** Many men have the attitude that work is their first priority and have a self-image that encourages a denial of illness to continue to be able to provide.
7. **Drop your shorts.** Men often have trouble discussing emotions, sexual problems, and mental health issues like depression. Again, finding a doctor you are comfortable with is key.

often itself cause impotence. On the flip side, the earlier you become aware of your vital signs—blood pressure, cholesterol, heart rate, blood sugar, and diet—the better chance you have of avoiding these conditions or being able to treat them through less extreme means.

Now I'm not talking about this to be shocking or sensational. The point is this: *Men, get thee to a doctor*. The time to think about the health of both your little guy and your big guy is *now*. It's not manly to get cancer. It's not manly to drop dead from a heart attack at fifty-two. It's not manly to be told you can't drink beer anymore because you've got diabetes. What's manly and sexy and appealing is to be strong, be healthy, and be there a long time to love the people who are important in your life.

How to Get a Man to the Doctor

Scare him. "Hey, has that spot on your back always been there?"

Go with him. One really is the loneliest number at the doctor's office.

Bribe him. Sexy outfit, candlelight, dinner without the kids. 'Nuff said.

Flatter him. "Have I ever told you how sexy you look in that little exam gown?"

Emotions Aren't Just for Women

Seventy percent of people who seek help for mental issues are women. It's not that you guys are any saner than women (hey, I heard that!), but that women are more likely to admit they need help and seek it out. But that's not to say that men don't have their own ways of coping. Men abuse alcohol and drugs three times as much as women do. Testosterone, or just "being a man," is often blamed for your reluctance to ask for help and instead act out in ways that are violent, aggressive, or harmful to yourself. Now anyone who's watched a group of boys and a group of girls playing wouldn't tell you for a second that men and women aren't created different—not better, not worse, just different.

But rather than just laying it at the feet of "being manly" or having too many hormones, most of how you learn to cope with feelings, stress, pressure, and the other facts of everyday life is from seeing how the adult men behave when you are a child, from how society portrays men on television and in movies, and from how other boys around you expect you to behave. And while many parts of dealing with your emotions from a more rational point of view are great, buttoning up your emotions when they become too overwhelming can have devastating effects on your health and your life. Men account for almost 75 percent of the deaths from suicide in the United States. And while often portrayed as a woman's condition, depression affects men just as hard.

Some of the emotional conditions that you should be on watch for include:

- **Anxiety** feelings of uneasiness, uncertainty, fear, and agitation
- **Panic** overwhelming feeling of flight-or-fight emotions that cause your heart to race, sweating, and feelings of dread
- **Depression** feelings of overwhelming sadness, hopelessness, and loss of interest in daily life and activities
- **Insomnia** an inability to get the sleep you need to fully function; can be both physical and mental
- **Bipolar disorder** (also called manic depression) rotating mood swings with severe highs (mania) and extreme lows (depression). You may feel completely normal in between.
- **Anger** feelings of frustration and turmoil that often lead to violent (physical and verbal) outbursts

If you begin to feel that you might be experiencing one of these conditions, the most important thing you can do is to go to an

How Stressed Out Are You?

	Always	Sometimes	Never
1. I get agitated when I feel people are wasting my time.	3	2	1
2. I drive fast, even when I'm not in a rush, and I get into arguments with other drivers.	3	2	1
3. I like to cram my schedule with more than I can do so that I don't waste a moment.	3	2	1
4. I think I'm the best person to be in charge of things because other people won't do the job as well.	3	2	1
5. I feel as if my relationships take me away from more important things that I need to get done.	3	2	1
6. I don't like to waste my time doing menial tasks like cleaning the house or working in the yard.	3	2	1
7. I have problems getting a good night's sleep because my mind is going a mile a minute all the time.	3	2	1
8. I get upset when other people do well, even if I'm doing well myself.	3	2	1
9. I am short with the people around me when they disappoint me or don't live up to my expectations.	3	2	1
10. I often feel tense and keyed up, but relax myself by drinking or taking medication.	3	2	1

Scoring and Evaluation

25–30 Warning! Warning! You seem to be putting yourself under a lot of stress. You are putting your health and well-being at risk by expecting too much from yourself and others. Stress management classes might help you relax.

15–25 You have stress in your life that could be affecting both your physical and mental health. Take a look at some ways you could slow down and enjoy life.

10–15 Everyone has stress in their life, but you seem to have it mostly under control. Stay on top of your stress to make sure it stays in check.

experienced professional for an evaluation and possibly treatment. These conditions are nothing to be ashamed of. In fact, admitting that you could use someone to take a look at you shows an enormous amount of strength. You might also feel more comfortable talking with a close friend or your spouse first. It's much better to get it off your chest and can even help those around you understand why you have been behaving toward them in a way that is unusual for you. And if you find yourself having thoughts of suicide, get medical help right away. There's a misconception that everyone thinks of killing themselves once in a while. While a fleeting thought in a moment of frustration may not be dangerous, thoughts of suicide accompanying a mental condition should be taken very seriously.

There are all kinds of treatments available for mental conditions, from talk therapy to medication to group therapy sessions. Refer to the "Mental Health Therapies" list in the resources section at the back of the book for some insight into how different therapies work and then find a professional whom you like, respect, and feel comfortable working with. And keep in mind that many emotional conditions are only temporary and can surface because of an event like the death of someone close to you, an illness, losing your job, or other stresses in your life. Getting treatment doesn't mean you're "weak" or "crazy." It just means you want to get back to being the best you that you can be.

Hello Mother, Hello Father

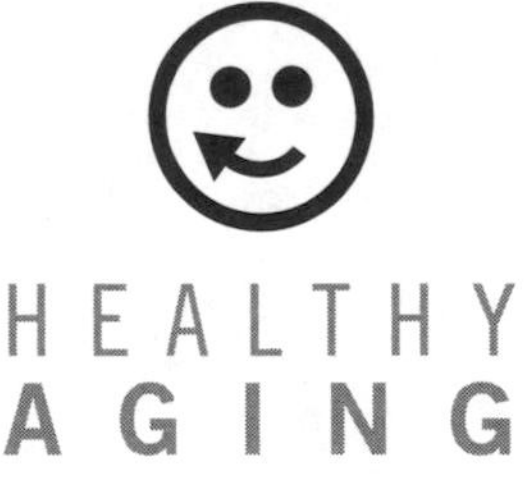

I think all of us would agree that the gigantic leap in life expectancy made in the last hundred years is fantastic. We're living longer, staying healthier, and enjoying our loved ones longer and longer. But let's face it, we're not altogether prepared for this growth in longevity, the growth in the population of older adults, and the issues our society faces from this change.

In fact, with the first wave of baby boomers starting to reach their sixties, most were anticipating a healthy, relatively comfortable ten to fifteen years of retirement. What some didn't expect is that while their kids are now mostly out of the house and on their own, instead of being free to think of golfing, traveling, and relaxing, many have a

Leaps in Life Expectancy

Neanderthal	20
Classical Greece and Rome	28
Medieval England	33
Late nineteenth century	37
Early twentieth century	50
Western world, 1940s	65
Western world, current	79

new responsibility awaiting them—caring for a spouse, a parent, or another family member.

Often, getting involved in the health and care of a loved one can bring an incredible amount of stress and discord into a family and onto the caregiver. Children, husbands, and wives resent the intrusion into their routines, and when you're trying to think of everyone's needs, something's got to give—typically the caregivers themselves. One study published by the National Academy of Sciences showed that the stress of caring for an Alzheimer's patient at home can prematurely age the immune system, putting the caregiver at risk for developing conditions like heart disease and even cancer. The study also showed that caregivers of those with a chronic condition ran a 63 percent greater chance of dying prematurely, causing researchers to label them the "second victims of Alzheimer's."

Add to this the inherent discrimination that exists in our health care system against older adults. Many health professionals demonstrate a lack of respect, a lack of care, and a lack of understanding of the health issues of aging patients. In a survey at Johns Hopkins University School of Medicine, 80 percent of students said they would admit a ten-year-old girl with pneumonia to intensive care and give her aggressive treatment, but only 56 percent said they would do the same for an eighty-five-year-old woman. Many doctors and other health care professionals think that medical problems in older patients are inevitable with age—"they're just getting older." Not only does this problem cost a lot of money by ignoring early treatment that could prevent conditions before they become serious threats, but it also forces more and more older Americans to become unnecessarily dependent on family members.

According to the Centers for Disease Control, nine out of ten adults over the age of sixty-five don't get the appropriate screenings and tests, including glaucoma, basic cancer, and even hearing loss tests. In addition, the poor treatment and lack of respect older patients receive when they attempt to get care means that many need to be accompanied by someone who can advocate for them, communicating with the doctors and demanding the respect they deserve—yet another responsibility for their caregivers.

Caring for Them, Caring for You

What can you do to make this easier on everyone, yourself included? Just as with kids, you're going to want to make sure that the person you are caring for has all of their vital health information available. Paramedics often describe how frustrating it is to enter a home for an emergency call, only to find family members standing over someone who is unconscious, with no information about their medical conditions, the medications they take (which is often quite a few), and who their doctors are. Emergency health care workers, including EMTs, doctors, and nurses, routinely have to administer life-saving procedures and medications under stressful, rapidly changing conditions and need the best, most complete information they can get to help them do their job and save your loved one's life.

Conditions That Often Go Untreated in Older Americans

- Incontinence
- Depression
- Dementia
- Vision or hearing loss
- Malnutrition
- Sexual dysfunction

Review your family members' health information with them to make sure that it's complete. Make sure it is written down and that everyone in the family knows where to find it. Even older adults who are in perfect health can find it hard to remember all of their medications, doctors, operations, tests they've had, and so on. When they come to the doctor's office or hospital prepared with all of their vital information, you'll be surprised at the difference in the quality of care they receive.

One man, Javier, told me that when he accompanied his mother to her doctor the first time, she wasn't able to answer most of the doctor's questions about her medications or her past medical history. "The doctor treated her like she was a child. You could see he was very impatient and frustrated. Looking at it from his end, we didn't seem to take his time very seriously because we weren't really prepared." Javier said that after that visit, he sat down with his mom and gathered all of her medical records and wrote down a chronological history of her operations and conditions. He also went through her medicine cabinet and made a list of everything that she was taking. "The next time we went to the doctor—same doctor—totally different experience. The doctor could tell that we took my mom's health very seriously and he seemed to be much more into finding a solution to what was bothering her. He looked over all of her prescriptions and actually got rid of two of her medications that she no longer needed—something that had really been bothering her. He also took

RESOURCE

Locate Your Papers

You can find an AARP form that will help families find their important documents at www.aarp.org/families/caregiving/caring_parents/valuable_documents.html.

5 minute clinic

6 Things to Take to the Next Doctor Visit

If you're taking Mom or Pop (or Auntie or Uncle) to the doctor, make sure they've got what they need.

1. **Symptomatic.** Take a written list of all symptoms, complete with dates and times.
2. **List of meds.** Write, write, write. The doctor needs to know exactly what drugs they're taking, including over-the-counter, herbals, and vitamins. You need to write them down because it is easy to forget one or two during an office visit.
3. **Historical significance.** Take a complete health history, especially if you are visiting a specialist for the first time who is not familiar with your loved one's situation.
4. **Million-dollar question.** Take a written list of questions that you want to ask the doctor. Most patients ask their questions when the doctor is finished and about to leave the room. This leaves little or no time to answer your questions. Be prepared and ask questions early.
5. **Pen and paper.** Directions on how to use a medication or how to follow a treatment plan have a higher chance of being effective if they are written down. Always write down instructions the doctor gives and verify with the doctor that you both understand them.
6. **You.** Don't let your loved ones go to office visits alone if they are uncomfortable or if you think that they might be unable to understand what the doctor is telling them. Sometimes emotions can keep someone from being objective in a stressful situation. A loved one or a friend can be an advocate to get the information they need and help them make decisions.

her complaints seriously and ended up sending her to see a specialist. It was like a transformation."

Caring for the needs of another adult, no matter who she is, can be a big responsibility and can place a great deal of stress on the caregiver, both physically and mentally. Take a few steps to get the help you need and make sure that the responsibility doesn't overwhelm you.

6 Ways to Care for Others without Losing Your Mind

You've heard the adage that you're no good to anyone if you're no good to yourself, and nowhere is it more true than when you're responsible for another person's emotional and physical needs. Caregivers' own health often deteriorates, putting themselves as well as the person they're caring for at risk. Be aware of when you are reaching your limits and need a break. Also, be careful of jeopardizing your relationships with your spouse, children, family, and friends. These relationships are what give you joy and they can be put under incredible strain by a caregiving relationship. Your children or spouse may resent the time you take away from them. Keep the lines of communication open so that everyone feels involved and engaged. Take some time to take care of yourself and understand what your limits and abilities are.

1. **Educate Yourself**

   Learn as much as you can about your loved one's

   - legal matters
   - health, life, and long-term care insurance
   - health conditions
   - financial situation

2. **Open Lines of Communication**

   Talk openly with your loved ones about their feelings and what they want. Be sure to express your own feelings and let your loved ones know that you will do your best to help them get the resources they need to feel cared for and loved.

3. **Involve the Whole Family**

   You can't do this alone. Use these strategies to get the help you and your loved ones need.

   - Hold a family conference including as many family members as possible.
   - Talk to your immediate family about why helping your loved one is important.
   - Ask everyone what they can do to help (money, time, housing).
   - Solicit ideas about outside help and get input from everyone so the burden is not just on you.

4. **Encourage Independence**

   Help your loved ones help themselves. Encourage them to retain as much control as possible and to be independent as often as possible. Help them make their own decisions and respect their wishes as often as possible.

5. **Pay Attention**

   Watch for the signs that someone needs help (see page 210). It may be difficult for older adults to admit they can no longer be independent or take care of themselves the way they used to. Making the adjustment from a parent in charge to asking for help can be nearly impossible, so you'll need to look for signs without them asking.

RESOURCE

Help for Caregivers

Hook up with local resources for eldercare assistance at www.eldercarelink.com.

6. **Explore Your Options for Help**

   You don't have to go it alone. There are many different arrangements for care, so explore the options until you find the solution that works best for you, your loved one, and other family members. Some alternatives to consider:

   - Home care services can visit a home to provide health and personal care.
   - Adult day care services are similar to day care for children and can be a great relief two or three days a week. They also provide activities and interaction with other adults, relieving isolation and building relationships.
   - Respite care nurses or aides can come into a home to give a full-time caregiver time off and are often available through your local Department of Social Services.
   - Assisted living communities provide great services for independent adults who need some assistance. Services like meals, maid, laundry, and nurses may be included in the rent.

How to Know When Someone Needs Help

Keep an eye out for these signs that a loved one could use your help.

- **Mental health:** Watch for confusion, mood swings, sadness, or disorientation or memory problems.
- **Physical health:** Look for weight loss or gain, vision or hearing problems, difficulty walking, or other symptoms.
- **Medication or alcohol use:** Be on guard for medication or alcohol abuse or dependency. Look out for difficulty remembering to take medications or managing dosages.
- **Grooming and personal habits:** Watch for a shift in bathing and dressing habits or the simple tasks of living. Are they able to drive safely, keep their house, go shopping, and prepare meals?
- **Safety:** Have they fallen prey to door-to-door or telephone schemes? Is their home unsafe or are they unable to safely maintain it? Are they fearful when traveling within their community? Watch for burns or other injuries that indicate physical impairments.
- **Friends and support:** Have they withdrawn from their friends and social situations? Do they seem lonely and lacking companionship and visitors? Becoming homebound and disengaging from interaction with family and friends can signal depression or other emotional or physical issues.
- **Joyful living:** Be on the lookout for a loss of the joy of living. Depression becomes more common as you get older. Do they still have hobbies and interests they enjoy? Do they have enriching interactions with grandchildren, other family, and people in general, or do they seem angry and bitter?

- Skilled nursing facilities provide twenty-four-hour care for those who have serious needs but do not require hospitalization.

Staying Sharp

One of our biggest concerns about growing older is the potential loss of mental ability. The fear of things that affect our mind like Alzheimer's, strokes, or other injuries looms large. Most of us just assume that as we grow older we will see a decline in our memory, mental abilities, the ability to learn new things, and our reasoning. But research is showing that this doesn't have to be the case.

Typically memory loss begins with short-term memory—often referred to as having a "senior moment." Short-term memory is how our brains remember information that we're using right now, like the four or five items you need from the store, a phone number you just looked up, or a thought you wanted to add to a conversation. Typically your short-term memory can hold around seven items. If you try to remember more than it can handle, the middle items will often be lost. Once something has been registered and retained, it then moves to your long-term memory—sort of like saving something to your computer's hard drive. Your long-term memory has an unlimited capacity to remember information. However, finding information in your memory—or what scientists call "retrieval"—can be more difficult the older you get. When you're trying to remember the name of that actor you saw in that movie . . . that's a retrieval problem. Your memory stored it, but the more information your brain has to search through, the tougher it can be to find—just like a messy computer desktop.

So how can you help your brain get more organized and improve your memory? Your brain uses "triggers" to help you remember certain things, including images, colors, tastes, touch, sounds, smells, emotions, and language. Practice using all of your senses when you're trying to remember something. Don't just memorize someone's name. Try and associate it with other things about that person—envision how he looks, picture his favorite food, or hear a certain word he uses. And since the brain often blocks out unpleasant memories, try to focus on a positive image. Here's some more tricks you can use no matter what your age, to help you improve your memory:

Thanks for the Memories

1. **Be a teacher:** Get the basic idea of what you're trying to learn and explain it to someone in your own words.
2. **Talk to yourself:** Saying things out loud will give you another cue to help your brain catalogue and retain the information.
3. **Do a five-minute review:** If you go over what you learned a second time for five minutes, your retention will be much higher.
4. **Acronyms:** Remember ROY G. BIV (red-orange-yellow-green-blue-indigo-violet—the colors of the rainbow)? This tried-and-true method really works. Be creative and come up with a word or a phrase to help you memorize a list.
5. **Singing:** When my son just couldn't remember our address (a kindergarten assignment), my mom taught him a song she made up—We live at 2-2-2-3 Hummingbird Lane (not my real address!)—and the whole family went around singing it for weeks. That song still comes to mind whenever someone asks me my address.
6. **Chunk it up:** If you have trouble remembering something long (like a phone number), chunk it up into smaller segments. 1237650111 can become (123) (7650) (111). If you've got a list of twelve items, divide it into three groups of four similar items.
7. **Memory helpers:** Don't just rely on the power of your mind—give it all the help you can. Use notes on your refrigerator, egg and watch timers, and planners. Ask friends and family to help you remember things, too. Using a note doesn't mean you're losing your memory—it just helps your brain search to find the right trigger.

RESOURCE

Check Out Fun Memory Exercises

Here's a nifty Web site that helps you build memory skills with the Memory Gym: www.memorise.org.

Staying mentally and physically fit throughout your life is the best way to protect not just your memory, but your emotional health and mental ability as well. Older people who exercise three or more times a week have been shown to have a 30-to-40-percent lower risk of developing Alzheimer's and other types of dementia. When it comes to your mind, it's a case of "use it or lose it." Studies show that people with high mental stimulation can have as much as a 46 percent decrease in their risk for dementia. The key, researchers have found, is to exercise different areas of your brain. This can be challenging as

15 Quick and Easy Brain Teasers

1. Solve a crossword puzzle.
2. Learn the words to a new song.
3. Memorize a poem.
4. Tutor a child.
5. Learn ten words in a new language.
6. Balance your checkbook—without a calculator.
7. Write a letter—use a pen and paper, not the computer.
8. Read the newspaper every day.
9. Debate an issue with a friend.
10. Make a list of the top-ten places you'd like to travel to.
11. Draw a cartoon.
12. Do a jigsaw puzzle.
13. Learn a new craft or a hobby.
14. Join a church, a community center group, or a card club.
15. Get a journal. Write down ten great things that happen to you every day—simple stuff counts!

we age since our natural tendency is to shy away from learning new things or going outside our comfort zones. Staying socially engaged—volunteering, joining a club, or taking a class—can be one of the best ways to keep your mind active and healthy. You need to engage in new activities and be stimulated by new people and challenges.

It's a Family Affair

Whether your family consists of just you, you and your spouse, children, or an extended family of brothers, sisters, aunts, uncles, and grandparents, the bottom line is that everyone should be more involved in their own health and the health of each and every family member. Your family is your core, the group of people who most affect your habits—what you eat, how active you are, your mood, your happiness, your joy. In order to make feeling good, being healthy, and living longer a priority for everyone in your family, it's essential that you open up the channels of communication and make it a topic for constant discussion.

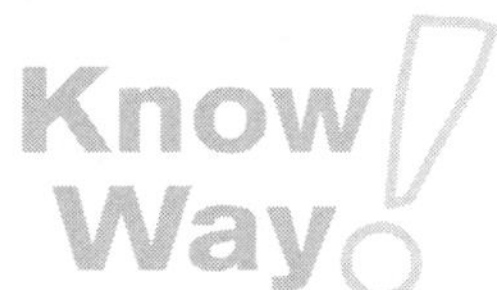

Think you're forgetful? A goldfish has a memory span of three seconds! Hey! I think I married one of those!

Taylor's Eighth Law of Health

Be healthy to live,
don't live to be healthy.

Prescription 7

Make a Change

The End of the Beginning

As you reach this seventh prescription, you begin a truly revolutionary journey. This book is sending you on a journey by giving you tools you can use to find a healthier, happier life. But your journey has just begun. You have reached the end of your new beginning as an empowered health consumer and now you're ready to fight for your life.

You have at your disposal the most advanced health care in history. Doctors have never had more knowledge and skill to keep us healthy and treat us when we're sick. Tools for preventing, diagnosing, and treating every kind of health condition have never been more powerful. The only power that has been missing is your power to understand and use these amazing tools when you need and want them. You can now look at your health through new eyes—informed eyes, empowered eyes, eyes that know the true value of your health and the health of those you love.

Worth the Fight

Once I returned home from a particularly rough business trip. I had flown to New York to meet with executives—at their request—from a major health care company to discuss developing a new diabetes education program for their customers. I sensed something was wrong when the first question posed by the company's ad agency rep was a skeptical, "Tell me just how this product will make people buy more of their product."

"It won't," I answered, starting to mentally add up the company money I had wasted on the plane tickets, a hotel, and cab fare for myself and two staff members. "It's a health education program," I managed to continue. "It's designed to help people manage their diabetes—it's not supposed to sell them anything." From the looks around the table, I realized that I would not be returning home in a flurry of triumph.

That night, at home, I drowned my sorrows in a warm bubble bath. My husband entered the bathroom with trepidation, trying to understand the reason for my foul mood. "I'm wasting my life," I told him. "I'm sitting there in a meeting with someone who's called the Director of Health Education, who's got a four-million-dollar budget, and who's not the least bit interested in educating anyone. If I had that job, I would do things that made a difference. But here I sit. Why am I wasting my life trying to convince these companies that people deserve better care?"

Expecting his usual support, or at least a kind word or two, I was shocked when my husband stiffly told me, "Stop feeling sorry for yourself. They're trying to sell something—that's what they do. That's why you never wanted that job. Wasting your life? You're trying to help people not die from a heart attack because they don't go to the hospital, not get cancer because

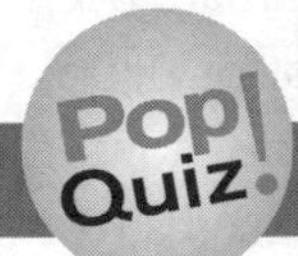

Smile for the Camera

1. Dogs have more teeth than humans. True False
2. People with gum disease are twice as likely to have a stroke or heart attack. True False
3. Bad breath is bothersome, but not a cause for concern. True False
4. Tooth enamel is the hardest substance in the body. True False
5. Philadelphia was the first city to add fluoride to its water supply. True False

Answers

1. True. People have thirty-two; dogs have forty-two. Score one for Fido!
2. True. Bacteria from your mouth can travel to your heart.
3. False. Bad breath can signal gum disease, tooth decay, strep throat, tonsillitis, sinusitis, and diabetes.
4. True. It is even harder than your bones.
5. False. Oakley, Idaho, gets that honor.

The definition of insanity is doing the same thing over and over and expecting different results.

—BENJAMIN FRANKLIN

they didn't get the right test soon enough, not lose a leg because they didn't understand how to manage their diabetes. You never did it because it was easy, you did it because you believed it was worth the fight. Frankly, I can't think of something that's less a waste of a life!"

Left alone to watch my bubbles pop one by one, I realized two things. One, my fingers were getting pruney, and two, he had a point. I mean, a husband's entitled to one, once in a while.

I don't tell you this story to trumpet myself as some kind of health hero, because I'm hardly that. I tell you because what you're setting out to do may not always be easy. You're going to face resistance—from your friends, from your family, from your doctor, from people selling you stuff, from the world around you. You're bucking a system that's been built up piece by piece over many years; a system that a lot of people have a lot of buy-in to keeping the same; a system where thousands of people die from mistakes every day and yet nothing seems to change; a system where your very life is at stake, yet no one's put you in charge.

But armed with what you now know, you're also going to find great doctors who want to help their patients. You're going to build a great circle of support within your family and friends. You're going to feel more control and more power, and you'll be better prepared to meet the health challenges that life brings your way.

You've got to fight for your life. You've got to make that commitment to yourself to take charge and live the healthiest life you can—not give up everything you enjoy, not become an exercise addict, not cringe in fear at every symptom. But live every day with the knowledge, power, and spirit to be the healthiest and happiest you can, making your own decisions and living your own life.

If you promise to do that for your family and yourself, I'll promise to keep fighting that fight. Because that's something worth fighting for.

It's in Your Hands

I think a lot of us may feel that our health happens *to* us. We go along, living our lives, minding our own business, and then one day, ewww . . . we don't feel so good. We go to the doctor, tell him our symptoms, have a few tests, and *bam!* The doctor tells us we've got whateveritis. "How did this happen?" we think. You know by now that I won't say that getting a condition or illness is your fault. It's not. But . . . take a look at a few recent headlines:

> RESEARCHERS IDENTIFY TOP FIVE RISK FACTORS THAT LEAD TO OVER ONE-THIRD OF CANCERS WORLDWIDE: OBESITY, LACK OF FRUITS AND VEGETABLES, PHYSICAL INACTIVITY, SMOKING, AND EXCESSIVE USE OF ALCOHOL
>
> STUDIES FIND MOST HEART RISK DUE TO BAD HABITS
>
> STUDY SAYS IMPROVING FITNESS MAY BOOST BRAIN POWER
>
> FINDINGS: NEARLY TWO-THIRDS OF THOSE WITH DIABETES AREN'T PROPERLY CONTROLLING THEIR BLOOD SUGAR

Looks as if, in many ways, we're happening to our health, not the other way around. The fact is, bird flu and anthrax and contaminated food aside, the biggest threat to our health may be . . . *us*! With the advancements our medical system has made in treating infectious diseases, injuries, and many life-threatening diseases, the real challenge today is how to deal with chronic conditions where much of the control is in the patient's hands. Doctors will tell you that healthstyle changes often affect the outcome of a patient's care more than any other medical treatments physicians have to offer. Your doctor can play a role in helping you make changes, but lots of doctors feel that urging patients to change doesn't seem to do much good. In *Changing for Good*, Jo Prochaska writes that only 20 percent of people who seek medical care are ready to change their behaviors.

In Canada, a man is three times more likely to have seen a doctor in the last year than a woman.

But let's stop blaming, and let's start changing. I'm not saying you can prevent everything, but let's face it, among the things that are the biggest threats to our lives and our well-being—heart attacks, cancer, stroke, diabetes—you've got the power to do little things that can make a big difference in your health and your life.

Ch-ch-ch-changes

"Yeah," you say, "but it's not so easy to change." Agreed. We humans are creatures of habit. We like things the way they are. Change can be tough. But let's look at why.

One of the big misconceptions about making a change is that failure is bad. In fact, researchers studying people who successfully gave up smoking found that the one thing they all had in common was

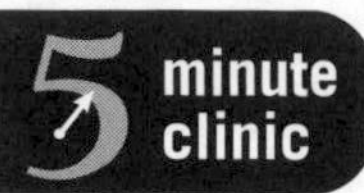

5 Tips for Getting through Withdrawal

Whether it's cigarettes, potato chips, coffee, or your cell phone, going without something is the most difficult part of making a change. Here are some strategies you can use to help you get through a craving.

1. **Stay calm.** Remember that craving your old habit is perfectly natural and normal and a necessary part of the cycle of change. So take a deep breath, relax, and remember, this too shall pass.
2. **Use the short-term delay method.** Don't think about not giving in permanently, just think in ten-minute increments. Think "I won't have a coffee for ten minutes, then I'll see how I feel," and do something distracting. After ten minutes, try the same tactic again. After a few sessions, it's likely your craving will have passed.
3. **Change your environment.** Whatever you're doing, wherever you are, change it as much as possible. If you're at a basketball game and feel like eating nachos because you see someone eating them down the aisle, get up from your seat and walk around the stadium (just not past the nacho stand). If you're watching TV and want to smoke, get up off the couch and go take a shower (you can't smoke in there!).
4. **Avoid giving in as long as possible.** Just remember that the craving will go away whether you give in or not. You won't crave french fries when you wake up in the morning, trust me.
5. **Drink some water.** Whatever you're longing for, water will (1) distract you, (2) fill you up, and (3) give you something to do with your hands so they can't be eating, smoking, or drinking.

that they had tried several times to quit before and had failed. It seems that the ability to get back up on the horse and try again is what makes change happen, not—as you might think—getting it right the first time. One of the great things about a failed attempt to make a change is that you can learn what trips you up and devise a strategy for overcoming that obstacle the next time you try.

Let's say you're trying to give up french fries. You go along fine until one day when you've got no time for anything—picking up the kids, going to the dentist, rushing to work. Finally it's eight o'clock in the evening and you haven't eaten anything all day, except for that half doughnut as you ran out the door. You're driving the kids home from soccer, and they're clamoring for fast food. You pull up to the drive-through because you're just too tired to cook. The kids place their orders for burgers and fries. You know it's better not to order anything and to grab something healthy at home, but what the heck, you yell out an order of large fries for yourself.

Well, there goes that change, right? Wrong. Let's look at the facts.

1. Your day was too busy to allow you to eat well.

2. You waited too long to eat and were starving.
3. You were too tired to make a healthy dinner for your kids or yourself.
4. You didn't have a healthy choice ready to make at the fast-food place.

These aren't huge mistakes and are certainly understandable given the circumstances of everyday life for most of us—too much to do, too little time, too little willpower! But instead of kicking yourself, you can take a few minutes to come up with a few counterstrategies so that next time you're ready. For example:

1. Take a good hard look at your and your kids' plates. I don't mean the ones the food is on, I mean how many things you try to do in a day. Everyone overschedules once in a while, but if you feel as if you regularly don't have the time to get something healthy to eat, you may want to reevaluate your schedule and see where you can make some time to take care of yourself.
2. Get some "fast-food" healthy snacks that you can carry around with you. Grocery stores have more and more of these now if you just look: carrots in single servings, 100-calorie snack packs, even—a radical idea—an apple!
3. Try to find some easy, healthier food alternatives for when you're really beat.
4. You know your kids are going to want fast food. You know they're going to scream so much that you'll eventually give in—at least once in a while. C'mon, you know you will. So take a few minutes to go online and look at the menus of their favorite places. Write down a couple of healthier options you can choose from so you're prepared when you go there.

Habits People Would Most Like to Change

- Poor diet
- No exercise
- Excessive drinking
- Aggressive driving
- Procrastinating
- Spending money
- Arguing
- Not getting enough sleep

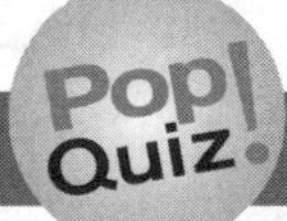

Is Your Food Safe?

1. What temperature should your refrigerator be set to?
   a. 55°F b. 45°F c. 40°F
2. What temperature should your freezer be set to?
   a. 32°F b. 20°F c. 0°F
3. To be thoroughly cooked, the internal temperature of poultry should be:
   a. 212°F b. 150°F c. 185°F
4. How long can you keep meat frozen?
   a. 2 months b. 4 months c. 6 months
5. Which way should meat not be thawed?
   a. refrigerator b. microwave c. at room temp

Answers

1. c 2. c 3. c 4. b 5. c

This is just one example, but it shows you how you can take a failure or falling off the wagon and turn it into knowledge you can use for your next try.

When it comes to your healthstyle habits, making a change can seem like an overwhelming project. We often go through our day thinking that our habits are just things that happen and not realizing that every food we eat, every step we take, every decision we make affects our bodies, our health, and our life span in some way. That's not to say you have to calculate every thing you do. The key is to identify some habits that you feel you want to change, determine what stage of changing you're in, and give yourself an easy way to make that change.

The Stages of Change

When you begin the journey toward making a change, there are several phases that you go through—probably without realizing it. We're going to take a look at each stage so that you can learn to recognize them and understand your feelings. Then I'll give you some strategies you can use to move yourself ahead to the next stage and onward to a new you!

1. What, Me Change?
2. Ping-Pong
3. I Think I Can
4. Lights, Camera, Action!
5. Keep Up the Good Work
6. Oops! I Did It Again

"What, Me Change?" Stage

In this stage you're not even considering a change or don't think you need to change. For example, when your doctor tells you that you have a prediabetes condition, your first instinct may be to deny that could ever be a problem. "No one in my family has ever had diabetes. Your test is screwed up or something. I'm not changing what I eat because of some stupid test." You're likely to be annoyed or defensive if someone even brings up the idea of you changing. You may have an underlying feeling that some of your habits aren't the healthiest, but believe that change will be too difficult and that "things are fine the way they are."

"What, Me Change?" Strategies

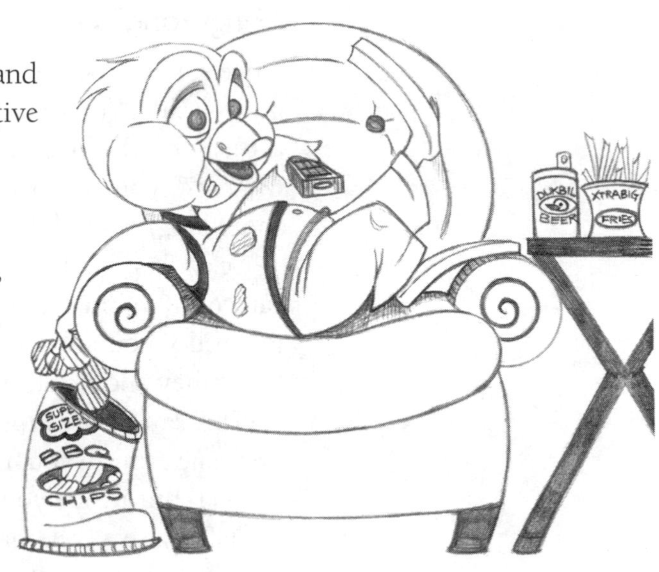

Try these strategies to move yourself forward and realize that you may want to make a positive change.

1. **Make sure your goals match your behaviors.**
   If you say "I want to live a long time" but deny that you should stop smoking, you might see a conflict between what you say and what you do.
2. **Educate yourself.**
   Find out what you can about conditions or habits you have and how they might affect your health or your life.

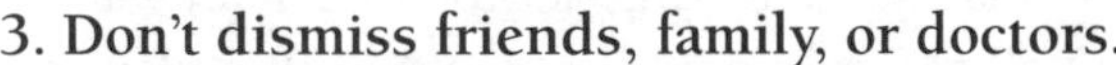

3. **Don't dismiss friends, family, or doctors.**
   Try to keep an open mind when those around you suggest a need for a change. Also consider the source, and check with someone else. If Mom tells you you're too skinny, ask your doctor if she thinks you're underweight or if Mom's just being Mom.

If You're in the "What, Me Change?" Stage

Questions to Ask Yourself

If people around you are suggesting to you that a change in a habit might be in order, but you just don't see it, ask yourself the following questions. If you have mostly "yes" answers, that might indicate that you indeed have a habit that is negatively impacting your health, your life, your work, or your relationships with others.

1. Do you respect the people who have suggested you might need a change?	Yes	No
2. Do you recognize that your habit is considered by others to be unhealthy?	Yes	No
3. Do you find yourself making excuses for continuing this habit?	Yes	No
4. Do you have difficulty picturing what your life might be like if you changed?	Yes	No
5. Does your habit interfere with your life, your job, your relationships, or your goals?	Yes	No

If you answered mostly "yes," you may be ready to move on to the "Ping-Pong" stage. ⇨

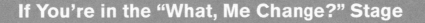

"Ping-Pong" Stage

Once you've acknowledged that your habit may be adversely affecting your life, you've moved to the "Ping-Pong" stage. This stage may actually be the one to cause you the most stress. If in "What, Me Change?" you say, "Hell no, I won't go!" here you say, "I should, I shouldn't, I should, I shouldn't"—just like a Ping-Pong ball.

Scientists say that most smokers in the United States fall into this category. On one hand, they want to continue to enjoy smoking and get mad when anyone brings up quitting. On the other hand, they know they should stop for hundreds of reasons.

This can be true for any habit that affects your health. You (and everyone around you, it feels like) might know that your habit is bad for you, but inside you are ambivalent about changing it. I remember talking to a colleague about whether she should give up coffee—it was wrecking her stomach and making her too hyper, and she knew she could do without all the caffeine. "I come up with a plan to stop drinking it, but what gets me every time is that I just really, really like it. I like the energy it gives me and I like how it tastes. I like stopping for a cup in the morning. I don't want to be someone who says, 'I don't drink coffee.'"

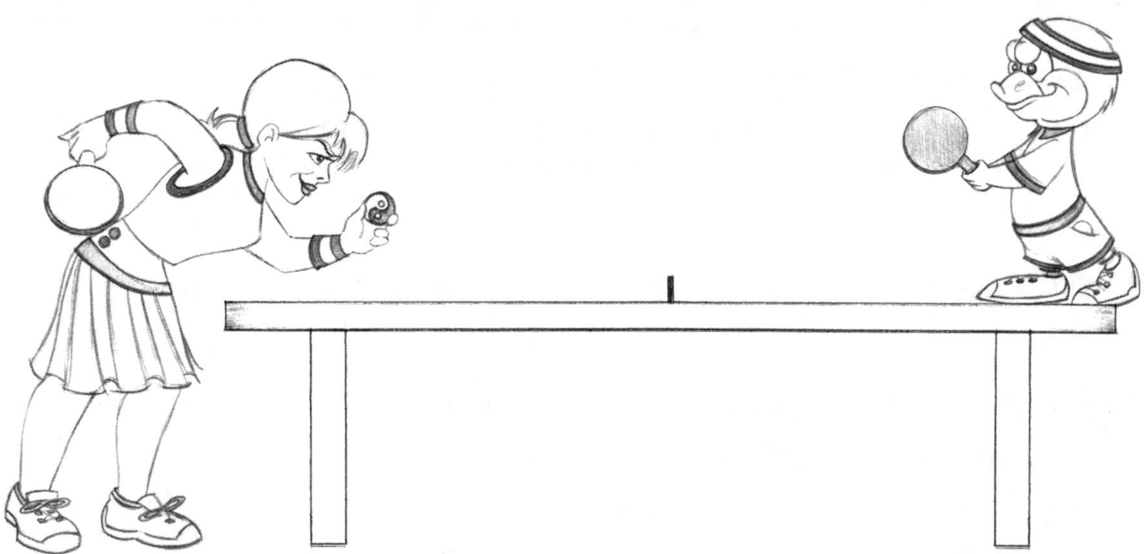

It's possible to stay in this stage for a long time—even years—while you bounce between wanting to change and not finding enough motivation.

"Ping-Pong" Strategies

These strategies can help you recognize your ambivalence and figure out how you can drive yourself closer to making a change.

1. **Accept your reluctance to change.**
   Doctors refer to this as "rolling with resistance." It's only natural.
2. **Make a pros-and-cons list.**
   Write down the reasons you want to make the change. But also write down the reasons you don't want to. It's okay to admit, "I really enjoy smoking." Acknowledging that fact will allow you to accept what you have to give up.
3. **Make a list of your past successes.**
   Think about things you have achieved that were hard. Try to find things in other areas of your life where you tackled tough jobs.

If You're in the "Ping-Pong" Stage

Questions to Ask Yourself

If you find yourself doing a lot of soul-searching about changing your habit, you're probably a Ping-Ponger. Asking yourself these questions will help you crystallize your commitment and decide if you're really ready to move forward.

1. Are there things about your habit that make you want to continue it?	Yes	No
2. Do you understand the reasons why you should change your habit?	Yes	No
3. Do you understand what you will be giving up if you make the change?	Yes	No
4. Can you picture improvements in your life if you change your habit?	Yes	No
5. Do you have other habits you've changed that you can use as a model?	Yes	No

If you answered mostly "yes," you may be ready to move on to the "I Think I Can" stage. ⇨

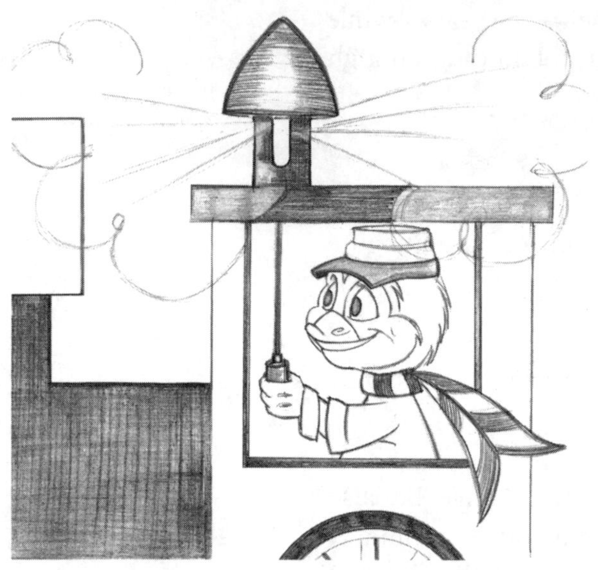

"I Think I Can" Stage

This stage is where you realize that you want to make a change and believe that you have the power and the will to do it. You're like the little engine that could, chuggin' up the hill: "I think I can, I think I can, I think I can, I think I can." Now's the time to ask yourself how strong your commitment is and what you're willing to do to make your change.

It's important now to really think through how you're going to make this change happen. Being dedicated is essential, but you also need to build yourself a road map of how you're going to get to your goal. Without a solid plan that includes the steps you're going to take, the resources you need, and the way you're going to overcome the obstacles when you get to them, you could find yourself with a lot of excitement about getting started, but wind up losing your motivation at the first little bump in the road.

"I Think I Can" Strategies

You'll also want to think about any help you need. One of the best places to start is with your doctor. For example, if your habit relates to exercise, she can give you a checkup to make sure there are no physical limitations. She can also point you to some exercise plans to get you started or tell you what other patients have done that worked for them. If your habit requires medication support (for example, treating depression or stopping smoking), seeing your doctor is a must.

It's a good time to start telling people about your plan, as well. You'll get their support and ideas, but you'll also push yourself to move forward with your change, since you've told everyone that you're going to do it.

1. **Make a plan.**
   Write down how you're going to make the change. Include the people and resources who can help you (such as family, friends, doctors, classes, and support groups).

If You're in the "I Think I Can" Stage

Questions to Ask Yourself

Making a change in your life isn't easy. It is very important to have a plan in place that includes strategies to help you overcome the obstacles you will inevitably face. Think about the worst possible scenario—you're giving up potato chips and your wife brings home a case of chips that someone gave her at the office. What will help you stick with your change and not give in?

1. Do you have a written plan with the steps you're going to take?	Yes	No
2. Do you have a list of the help you'll need—people, resources, information?	Yes	No
3. Do you know the obstacles you might run into while making your change?	Yes	No
4. Do you have a strategy to overcome each expected obstacle as well as the unexpected ones?	Yes	No
5. Have you talked to people about your plan to get their help, support, and ideas?	Yes	No

If you answered all "yes," you are ready to move on to the "Lights, Camera, Action!" stage. ⇨

2. **Come up with a solution for each obstacle.**
   Writing them down beforehand will keep you from getting caught off guard. If your change is to get thirty minutes of physical activity every day, what happens if it rains? Do you have an activity you can do indoors? You don't want a little shower to blow your entire plan!
3. **Tell others about your plan.**
   Tell lots of people about your plan. The more you brag it up, the more you'll get support (and, okay, maybe a little embarrassment) to keep going. But the support (and even the embarrassment) will go a long way toward helping you stick to your plan.

"Lights, Camera, Action!" Stage

Here's where the rubber hits the road. "Lights, Camera, Action!" is the stage where you put your plan to work. This is when the going can get tough—and when you'll need the most support from doctors, family, and friends. Depending on the size of your change (quitting smoking, for example), you may want to make an appointment with your doctor just to go over how things are going (and to get some encouragement). Expect it to be hard—it's going to be at first. You're

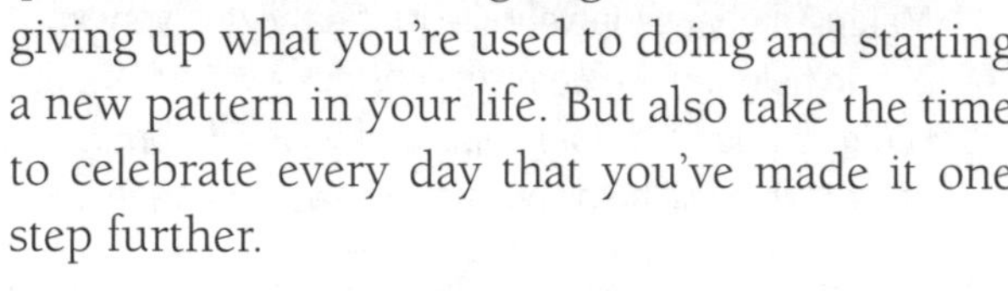

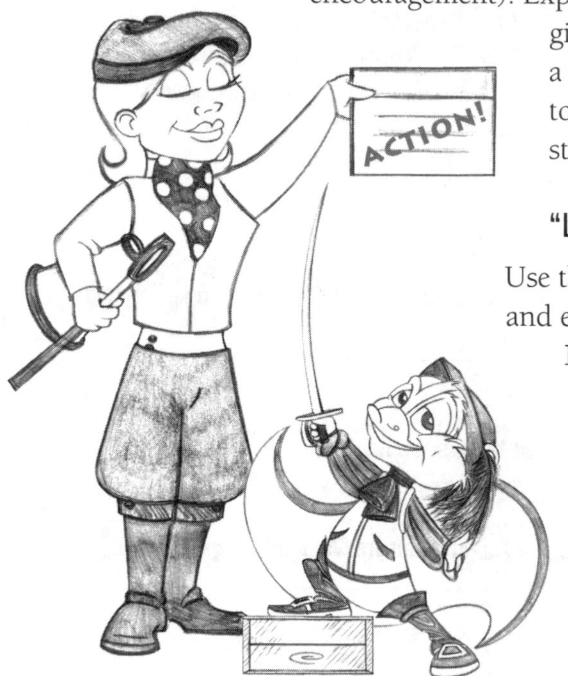

giving up what you're used to doing and starting a new pattern in your life. But also take the time to celebrate every day that you've made it one step further.

"Lights, Camera, Action!" Strategies

Use these strategies to help you stick with your plan and evaluate how you're doing.

1. **Use a journal.**
   Write down how you feel about the change and where you've had problems sticking to your plan. When you start to think about going back to your old habit, whip out your journal and write it down. It might sound silly, but just doing that will take your mind off it and help you come up with some strategies to overcome whatever obstacle you've reached.
2. **Call on your support group.**
   Here's where the resources you listed in your "I Think I Can" stage come in handy. Whether it's a friend, a family member, your doctor, a support group, even a book or other resource—go to them to get encouragement to make your change stick.
3. **Evaluate your plan constantly.**
   Don't think that just because you came up with a plan, it can't change. It should and will. There are going to be things you didn't anticipate. Instead of letting them turn you around, update your plan to face them. For example, if you're trying to quit smoking, you might not have thought about wanting a cigarette when you're driving. You get in your car, see that ashtray, and don't have a strategy to deal with it. Instead of falling back, get out of the car and take a few minutes to regroup. Think about

Change Works

Does changing your habits really make a difference? Over 140,000 lives of men in the United States have been saved since 1991 because they gave up smoking, reports the American Cancer Society. Now *that's* a reason to change!

If You're in the "Lights, Camera, Action!" Stage

Questions to Ask Yourself

This stage may last quite a while, so don't be in a rush to move on. The key to making a change is that it become a natural part of your daily life. That doesn't mean you don't think about how much you'd like to eat a big sticky bun once in a while—that's not going to happen for a long time. But it does mean that your life goes on with your new habit, rather than feeling the loss of your old one.

1. Do you feel good about having stuck with your change?	Yes	No
2. Has your change become a new part of your daily routine?	Yes	No
3. Did you accomplish the main parts of your plan?	Yes	No
4. Did you face any obstacles that you had to overcome and were you prepared?	Yes	No
5. Have you talked to people about your plan to get their help, support, and ideas?	Yes	No

If you said mostly "yes," you may be ready to move on to the "Keep Up the Good Work" stage. ⇨

what you can do—ask someone to remove the ashtray and lighter for you, find a CD you can sing to, or get a cup of coffee. Rework your plan instead of just jumping back into your old habits.

"Keep Up the Good Work" Stage

Phew! You made it. You've gone thirty days with your change and you're free and clear—out of the woods, home free, mission accomplished, done deal. Whoops—wait a minute—not quite. Okay, take a deep breath; stay calm, here goes . . . "Keep Up the Good Work" can be even harder than "Lights, Camera, Action!" *What*? All that suffering, all that work, and now maintaining your new habit is harder? Well, think about a big one—losing weight. A lot of people can lose weight. They radically change what they eat for a month or two or six. The weight drops off. They buy new clothes—"All right, I'm stylin'." But then they say, "I've lost this weight, I can give myself a little treat

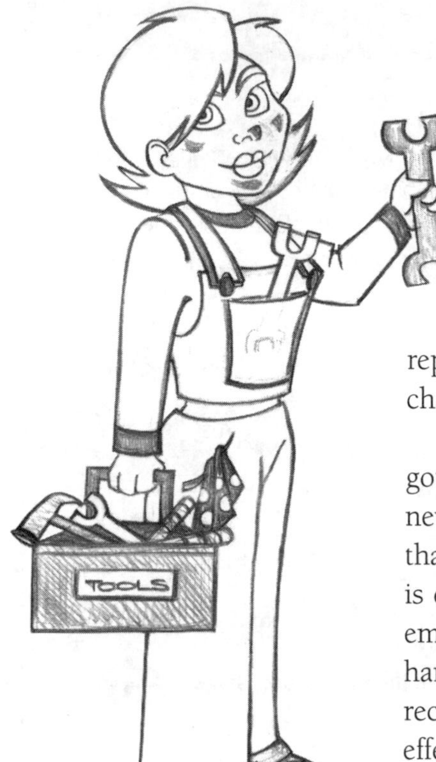

now and then, right?" One treat turns into two, two turns into five, which turns right back into their old eating habits or worse. That's why people who *diet*, rather than truly changing their eating habits, actually tend to gain more weight over time.

It's very frustrating, I know. You're trying to make a change and then *bam*! It backfires on you. That's why it's so important to make changes a little at a time so you can really incorporate them into your life and replace those old habits with new ones, rather than trying to change everything all at once.

During the "Keep Up the Good Work" stage, you've really got to embrace the change and make sure that it has become a new habit. It's also important to recognize that you can miss that old habit for months, even years. Maintaining your habit is especially critical when you go through a time of stress or emotional struggle. It's also good to admit that sometimes it's hard to stick with your change. That's when it's important to recall the joy you felt at making the change and the positive effect it's had on your life.

"Keep Up the Good Work" Strategies

1. **Have a maintenance plan.**
   Just as you planned for your change—now plan for your maintenance. What will you do if you feel like going back? Who can you talk to about it? What happens when you encounter a whole new situation that you hadn't counted on (such as a new job or a new girlfriend)?
2. **Make a list of the signs of a slip-up.**
   Think about the signals that you're going back to your old habit. Making a list will help you recognize them and be ready to deal with them.
3. **Keep celebrating.**
   Don't just let it lie. Remind yourself often of your success with a little celebration to keep reinforcing your positive change!

If You're in the "Keep Up the Good Work" Stage

Questions to Ask Yourself

Maintaining your change can be even harder than making it in the first place (just what you didn't want to hear, huh?). It's easy to get motivated and excited in the beginning, then, after your initial excitement, slowly slip back into your old habit: "I'll just pig out this weekend, then go back to my good eating on Monday." It happens; just be sure to watch for the signs that it's not a one-time splurge and your old habit is coming back to haunt you.

1. Do you have a plan to maintain your success?	Yes	No
2. Have you made it through any rough times and stuck to your change?	Yes	No
3. Do you know the signs that you are slipping back into your old habit?	Yes	No
4. Do you have a plan to resist that slide and get back on track?	Yes	No
5. Have you celebrated your success?!!	Yes	No

If you answered mostly "yes," *Congratulations!* You may *not* be ready to move on to the "Oops! I Did It Again" stage!!

"Oops! I Did It Again" Stage

> The best-laid plans of mice and men often go awry.
>
> —ROBERT BURNS

Okay, you knew it might happen. The quote to the right—well known from its use in the title of the John Steinbeck novel *Of Mice and Men*—refers to a little mouse in a poem by Robert Burns whose carefully plotted field gets plowed over by a farmer, demonstrating how many of our plans get mowed over by forces we can't control. Sometimes it happens. Even if you've thought it through, committed to your change, and executed it beautifully, relapses happen. Actually, they happen quite a lot.

Often you'll feel guilty or ashamed that you went back to your old behavior. "Gee, thanks," you'll mutter. "You set me up to tell everyone about my change, talk about my success, and now I've failed and look foolish." Actually, it's just the opposite. The people who look foolish are the ones who never try to change.

We've got a funny idea about failure. We believe, despite all evidence to the contrary, that failure is the opposite of success, when

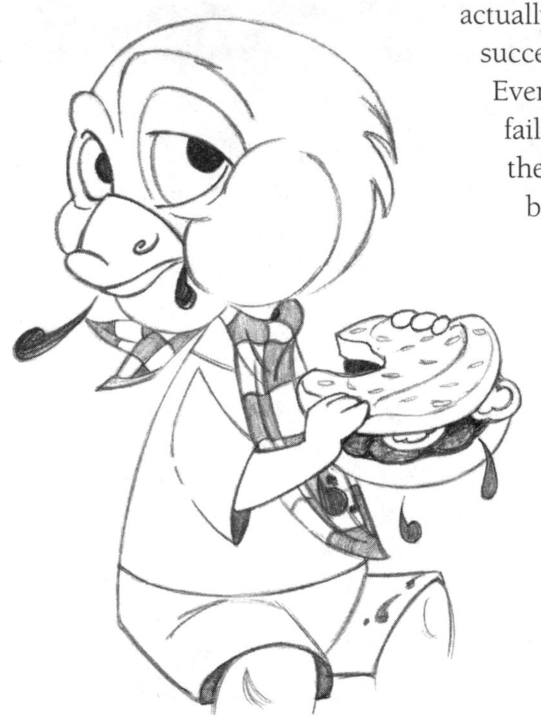

actually it's a necessary part. It's nearly impossible to have success without first having (usually many) failures. Even the people whose success we take for granted failed. Not once, not twice, but multiple times. And they didn't fail in secret. Many times the best and brightest suffer very public failures. The key is knowing that failure is going to happen, expecting it to happen, and not being embarrassed, dejected, or quick to give up when it does. In fact, the sooner you get done with your first failure, the sooner you'll be on the path to success!

Every success story you read is laced with anecdotes of failed attempts, utter desperation, and one defining trait—the ability to overlook the negative, the naysayers, and the problems and get back up on that horse. Keep in mind that you can't have a relapse unless you've first had success. A relapse isn't a reason to quit. It's one more reason to try again.

Famous Failures

Michael Jordan was cut from his high school basketball team.

Winston Churchill failed sixth grade.

Walt Disney was fired because he had "no good ideas."

Beethoven's music teacher told him he was hopeless.

Albert Einstein was advised to drop out of school because he would never amount to anything.

Henry Ford's first two auto businesses went bust.

"Oops! I Did It Again" Strategies

1. **Expect it.**
   This doesn't mean that you set yourself up for failure. You don't know which try is going to be the one that takes. But by realizing it might happen, you won't get too discouraged and will be even more willing to try again.
2. **Give up the guilt and the shame.**
   Get over yourself! Everyone fails, and like Walt Disney and Michael Jordan, you've now joined a pretty special club. If someone around you is discouraging, eject them from your Circle of Positivity! Use that as encouragement to "show them next time."
3. **Learn from it.**
   A relapse is a great time to look at what worked and what didn't and explore how soon you will be ready to try again.

If You're in the "Oops! I Did It Again" Stage

Questions to Ask Yourself

Okay, you slipped up. It isn't the first time someone's done it, and it won't be the last. You're disappointed and maybe feeling a little guilty, but why not take those emotions and channel them into motivation to try again? It's important that you honestly examine what happened (don't make excuses, take responsibility) and figure out how to keep it from happening again.

1. Do you understand why you went back to your old habit?	Yes	No
2. Do you still understand the benefits of your new habit?	Yes	No
3. Do you have the support you need to attempt your change again?	Yes	No
4. Do you have a plan that takes into consideration why you went back this time?	Yes	No
5. Do you have the motivation and the energy to try to make your change again?	Yes	No

If you answered mostly "yes," you may be ready to move back to the "I Think I Can" stage. 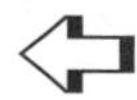

Thirty Days to a New You

Can you change your life in just thirty days? Well, maybe not your whole life, but how about one habit? Don't believe it? Pick one small habit you'd like to change. Stop eating french fries; drink four glasses of water a day; watch only one hour of TV a night; take the stairs at work instead of the elevator. Think of something you've always wanted to change and then come with me on a short but powerful journey. Make a copy of the 30-Day Pledge on page 233. Fill in your starting date—start on the first day of the month if you can. Any date will do, but for most of us it just feels better starting on 1. Now write down your habit. Here are some tips:

The *Able* Rules for Making Your Habit Stick

You'll be *able* to keep your new habit if you follow these rules!

- Keep it **SIZEABLE**. Your new habit has to have a size. "Eating better" is a good intention, but it's too vague. Instead, give it a size you can measure: "Eat five fruits and veggies every day." Now that's a killer new habit (not literally!). This way, you'll wake each day knowing exactly what you have to do to make your habit happen.

- Keep it **REASONABLE**. Do you know how you're going to make your habit a reality? Make sure there is a reasonable way to put your habit into action. If you say you're going to limit your calories to 1,500 a day, make sure you have an exact list of foods you're going to eat to keep you within that limit. If you can't come up with a list of foods, your habit may not be reasonable and may need to be adjusted.
- Keep it **MEASURABLE**. How will you know if you are sticking with your habit? Even if it just means a little notebook where you jot something down or carrying four pennies in your pocket and transferring one to an empty pocket each time you have a cup of coffee to limit your caffeine—whatever your method, measuring will help you track your progress to keep going.
- Keep it **DOABLE**. Be sure you have a way to overcome the inevitable obstacles. If you don't think about how you will handle temptation, habits, sabotage, or other obstacles, you won't be able to stick with your habit.

And most importantly, don't commit for more than thirty days. One of the biggest reasons people don't stick with diets is that they can't accept big, lifelong changes. The thought of never eating ice cream or steak or potatoes, *ever again*, is just too discouraging.

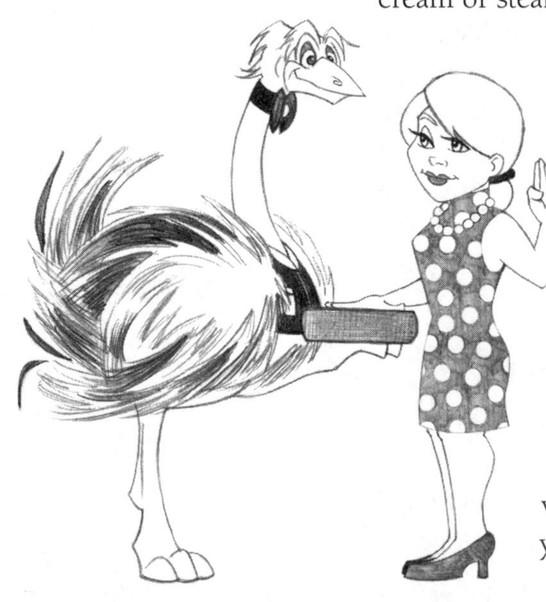

Now take the 30-Day Pledge that you've filled out to make a promise to yourself that you will commit for thirty days. I mean, you can do almost anything for thirty days, right? Pin your pledge on your refrigerator, your bulletin board, or your bathroom mirror—anywhere you'll see it every day. Each day that you successfully complete your goal, put a star in the box for that day. If you slip back on a day, mark that with an X. This will let you see your progress and encourage you to stick with your habit and fill up that chart with stars!

What you'll find, studies show, is that if you can stick with that habit for thirty days, it will actually become your new habit. Oh, you might still crave that french fry

30-Day Pledge

I, ______________________________, pledge for the next thirty days to
your name

commit to make the following change in my Healthy Life.

My New Habit:

____

____

____

____

____

____

____

Signature ______________________________ Date ________________

Witness (optional) _______________________ Date ________________

You'll be *able* to do it if you keep your new habit

- Sizeable
- Reasonable
- Measurable
- Doable

Progress Report

My start date ________________________

1. Fill in a ★ for each day you stuck to your new habit.
2. Place an ✘ in the box if you skipped your new habit.
3. Try again tomorrow!

Record Your Results

Number of ★ _____

Number of ✘ _____

You Did It!

Give yourself a round of applause! You made it through the month with your new habit. *You did it!* If you had a few missteps, don't worry, just try again!

once in a while (and even eat some), but your new reality will be a life without french fries. What will happen in those thirty days is that you'll find something to substitute for those fries. The key is to make sure your substitution is healthier! You'll no longer be in the habit of eating them, and my guess is that you won't even miss them too much anymore.

Now, your new french-fryless state may seem trivial, a small drop in the bucket of habits that you'd like to change. But attack a different habit every month for a year and what do you have? Twelve new habits! That's an incredible accomplishment. Imagine the changes you can make over five years!

That's sixty changes.

That's a new life.

Now here's a way to really kick it up a notch. Beginning on page 235, you'll find your Twelve-to-Life Plans. Pick a new habit for each month. I've given you a few suggestions, but pick a habit that's right for you. Write down your habit and use *able* criteria to make sure you're able to achieve your goal. Use your 30-Day Pledge for each new habit, and you're off and running!

My Twelve-to-Life Plan: January (Sample)

New Habit for January *Cut coffee back to only two cups per day*

☐ **Sizeable** What is the size of your new habit?

Two cups a day

☐ **Reasonable** How can it be done?

I will have one cup in the morning and one after lunch.

☐ **Measurable** How will you know you are sticking with it?

I will give myself two tokens. When I've used both, that's it!

☐ **Doable** How will you overcome obstacles?

I will substitute caffeine-free tea for coffee.

Action Steps

- *Find tokens*
- *Find teas I enjoy—stock up!*
- *Discard all coffee at home*
- *Talk to doctor about caffeine withdrawal*

Ideas for January

- Cut back caffeine
- Eat five veggies a day
- Get an annual checkup
- Stretch twice a week
- Have salad with dinner four nights a week

Your Ideas

____

____

____

____

My Twelve-to-Life Plan: January

New Habit for January ______________________________

☐ **Sizeable**	What is the size of your new habit?	
☐ **Reasonable**	How can it be done?	
☐ **Measurable**	How will you know you are sticking with it?	
☐ **Doable**	How will you overcome obstacles?	

Action Steps
- ______________________
- ______________________
- ______________________
- ______________________

Ideas for January
- Cut back caffeine
- Eat five veggies a day
- Get an annual checkup
- Stretch twice a week
- Eat salad for dinner four nights a week

Your Ideas

____

____

____

____

My Twelve-to-Life Plan: February

New Habit for February ______________________________

☐ **Sizeable**	What is the size of your new habit?	
☐ **Reasonable**	How can it be done?	
☐ **Measurable**	How will you know you are sticking with it?	
☐ **Doable**	How will you overcome obstacles?	

Action Steps
- ______________________
- ______________________
- ______________________
- ______________________

Ideas for February
- Hug your spouse daily
- Exercise three times weekly
- Don't add salt to food
- Give up or reduce candy
- Switch to lo-cal salad dressing

Your Ideas

____

____

____

____

(continued)

My Twelve-to-Life Plan: March (continued)

New Habit for March ______________________________

☐ **Sizeable** What is the size of your new habit?

____

☐ **Reasonable** How can it be done?

____

☐ **Measurable** How will you know you are sticking with it?

____

☐ **Doable** How will you overcome obstacles?

____

Action Steps
- ______________________________
- ______________________________
- ______________________________
- ______________________________

Ideas for March
- Eat beans once a day
- Take a walk every day
- Get preventive screenings
- Go to sleep one hour earlier
- Meditate for fifteen minutes every day

Your Ideas

____

____

____

____

My Twelve-to-Life Plan: April

New Habit for April ______________________________

☐ **Sizeable** What is the size of your new habit?

____

☐ **Reasonable** How can it be done?

____

☐ **Measurable** How will you know you are sticking with it?

____

☐ **Doable** How will you overcome obstacles?

____

Action Steps
- ______________________________
- ______________________________
- ______________________________
- ______________________________

Ideas for April
- Eat in four dinners/ week
- Eat four fruits a day
- Climb stairs every day
- Be nice to everyone
- Don't watch TV three days/week

Your Ideas

____

____

____

____

My Twelve-to-Life Plan: May

New Habit for May ______________________________

☐ **Sizeable** What is the size of your new habit?

____

☐ **Reasonable** How can it be done?

____

☐ **Measurable** How will you know you are sticking with it?

____

☐ **Doable** How will you overcome obstacles?

____

Action Steps

- ______________________________
- ______________________________
- ______________________________
- ______________________________

Ideas for May

- Write a positive affirmation every day
- Drink eight ounces water every day
- Do strength exercise three times a week
- Get up an hour earlier
- Don't eat snacks during TV

Your Ideas

____

____

____

____

My Twelve-to-Life Plan: June

New Habit for June ______________________________

☐ **Sizeable** What is the size of your new habit?

____

☐ **Reasonable** How can it be done?

____

☐ **Measurable** How will you know you are sticking with it?

____

☐ **Doable** How will you overcome obstacles?

____

Action Steps

- ______________________________
- ______________________________
- ______________________________
- ______________________________

Ideas for June

- Eat only whole-grain bread
- Try a new fruit every day
- Walk 10,000 steps each day
- Do aerobic exercise three times a week
- Eliminate one source of stress every week

Your Ideas

____

____

____

____

(continued)

My Twelve-to-Life Plan: July (continued)

New Habit for July ________________________________

☐ **Sizeable** What is the size of your new habit?

____

☐ **Reasonable** How can it be done?

____

☐ **Measurable** How will you know you are sticking with it?

____

☐ **Doable** How will you overcome obstacles?

____

Action Steps
- ________________________________
- ________________________________
- ________________________________
- ________________________________

Ideas for July
- Play ball with the kids twice a week
- Swim three times a week
- Cut out sugary snacks
- Do yoga twice a week
- Read a book a week

Your Ideas

____

____

____

____

My Twelve-to-Life Plan: August

New Habit for August ________________________________

☐ **Sizeable** What is the size of your new habit?

____

☐ **Reasonable** How can it be done?

____

☐ **Measurable** How will you know you are sticking with it?

____

☐ **Doable** How will you overcome obstacles?

____

Action Steps
- ________________________________
- ________________________________
- ________________________________
- ________________________________

Ideas for August
- No fast food
- Eat low-fat, low-sugar cereal for breakfast daily
- Practice "kind" driving
- Eliminate all soda
- Do twenty-five sit-ups a day

Your Ideas

____

____

____

____

My Twelve-to-Life Plan: September

New Habit for September ______________________________

☐ **Sizeable** What is the size of your new habit?

____

☐ **Reasonable** How can it be done?

____

☐ **Measurable** How will you know you are sticking with it?

____

☐ **Doable** How will you overcome obstacles?

____

Action Steps
- ______________________________
- ______________________________
- ______________________________
- ______________________________

Ideas for September
- Walk your children to school three days a week
- Turn off the cell phone in the car
- Play tennis twice a week
- Eat two apples a day
- Drink tea three times a day

Your Ideas

____

____

____

____

My Twelve-to-Life Plan: October

New Habit for October ______________________________

☐ **Sizeable** What is the size of your new habit?

____

☐ **Reasonable** How can it be done?

____

☐ **Measurable** How will you know you are sticking with it?

____

☐ **Doable** How will you overcome obstacles?

____

Action Steps
- ______________________________
- ______________________________
- ______________________________
- ______________________________

Ideas for October
- Do one random act of kindness every week
- Snack on raw veggies
- Ride your bike twenty minutes a day
- No potato chips
- Banish negative thoughts

Your Ideas

____

____

____

____

(continued)

My Twelve-to-Life Plan: November (continued)

New Habit for Novermber ____________________

☐ **Sizeable** What is the size of your new habit?

____

☐ **Reasonable** How can it be done?

____

☐ **Measurable** How will you know you are sticking with it?

____

☐ **Doable** How will you overcome obstacles?

____

Action Steps
- ____________________
- ____________________
- ____________________
- ____________________

Ideas for November
- Walk your mall five times
- No prepared food with sugar, fructose, or corn syrup
- Do family health history
- Say no to one request
- Give up french fries

Your Ideas

____

____

____

____

My Twelve-to-Life Plan: December

New Habit for December ____________________

☐ **Sizeable** What is the size of your new habit?

____

☐ **Reasonable** How can it be done?

____

☐ **Measurable** How will you know you are sticking with it?

____

☐ **Doable** How will you overcome obstacles?

____

Action Steps
- ____________________
- ____________________
- ____________________
- ____________________

Ideas for December
- Have a family fun night once a week
- Limit alcohol to twice a week
- Jump rope daily
- Compliment someone daily
- Don't put sauce on sandwiches

Your Ideas

____

____

____

____

Be Healthy to Live

So I know you've been wondering: Why is the final Health Law "Be healthy to live, don't live to be healthy"? I'll tell you why. People ask me all the time, because of what I do for a living, if I'm a "health nut." The answer is no. I have a very busy life—kids, husband, work, lecturing, writing, traveling, having fun (what's that last one again?). I want to be healthy, but I don't let it consume my life—I don't have the time for that. Good health is worth nothing without good friends, a loving family, rewarding work, and good times to enjoy. Don't let your health overwhelm you, even when it's overwhelming. My hope for this book is that you can get something out of it, feel more empowered about your health, and get some tools to help you deal better with your doctors, hospitals, and other health care providers. Then put the book down, get out there, and be happy and live your life to the fullest.

That's what's great about your health—you've got the rest of your life to get it right.

The Gift of a Day

A friend of mine who does not yet have children once said to me, "You talk so fondly of your children, you make it seem just so wonderful to have children."

My answer surprised him. "Yes and no," I said. "Don't get me wrong, having children was the single most joyful thing that's happened in my life. But until you have them, you don't realize how much sadness that joy also brings."

"Why sadness?" my friend wanted to know.

"Sadness because you know that someday they will be off on their own. Someday they will feel pain. Someday, by some circumstance, you will have to say good-bye. And knowing that, knowing that the day will come eventually no matter what you do, is a sadness I can't even explain to you. It's not that I don't enjoy every day. I've loved every single minute of raising my kids. I look forward to every phase of their life because every age brings such great new growth and wonder and fun. But when you become a parent, the secret that no one's told you is that by feeling such joy, such happiness, such love, you now know what true sadness can be."

"Wow, I never thought of it that way. Is it worth having children, knowing that one day you'll experience that sadness?"

Those of you with children know the answer: "Of course." When you love your children, you recognize a universal truth. You've been given a truly miraculous gift. The gift of today. The gift of learning to enjoy every day, every hour—not to squander a single second. You can't always let your worries go, but I'll tell you, when you look into the face of your child laughing, you see what life is really all about. It's that moment, that window, that joy. Not worrying about tomorrow, but letting go and loving each day you have with your child.

And that's what it seems we all have. We all have problems, aches, illnesses, pains, discomforts. Let's face it, some days just stink. Sometimes you even wonder, Who thought this up? We're born; we grow, grow, grow. We work, we get older, and then, just when we seem to have it figured out, our bodies start to rebel. But really, what we have is today.

Today. In reality, every day is what it's supposed to be. It's perfect, because every day we have is a wonderful gift. Even with all our imperfections, maladies, aches, and pains—a perfect day. The gift of a day. So take the steps you can to have the healthiest, longest, happiest life you can. Then let go and live your life.

I wish you all a healthy life filled with the gift of many days.

Be well.

Taylor's Ninth Law of Health

Every new day is a new chance to get it right.

Prescription 8

Be Healthy Every Day

Feeling better, living longer, and being healthier doesn't come from a sudden lightning bolt of activity. You can't go to the doctor, have every test under the sun, and think, "There. I'm good for another ten years." And we've all made that New Year's resolution to begin a big exercise program that falls by the wayside by January 10.

With every rising of the sun, think of your life as just begun.

—ANONYMOUS

Truly taking control of your health means finding a way to make healthy choices and feel better every day. On the following pages you'll find fifty-two weeks of healthy habits to get you started. They range from making healthier choices in what you eat to ramping up your physical activity level to sorting out your medications to getting ready for emergencies. Some are small things that can make a big difference, like switching to 2 percent milk, while others cover a bigger scope, like reviewing all your medications with your doctor.

Try out one tip a week for the next year. Just think how much better you'll feel after a year of healthier choices.

Good luck and good health!

52 Weeks of Health

1. **Drink at least one glass of 1 percent or 2 percent milk every day.**
   Whole milk gets 50 percent of its calories from fat, while 2 percent milk gets 35 percent and 1 percent milk gets 22 percent from fat. You'll barely notice the change in taste when you switch from whole milk. You'll get the great health benefits of added calcium and nutrients—great for men, women, and kids—without the calories of whole milk.

2. **Know your "big five" numbers.**
   Find out what your numbers are for the big five: (1) weight, (2) blood pressure, (3) cholesterol, (4) heart rate, and (5) blood sugar. If your numbers fall outside your healthy range, work with your doctor on a plan to get them under control. Buy a home blood pressure monitor so you can take your blood pressure regularly and keep track of the results.

3. **Learn CPR.**
   If someone you love experiences cardiac arrest, they are twice as likely to survive if you or someone else can begin CPR. CPR starts a "chain of survival" that delivers oxygen-rich blood to vital organs. CPR training will also teach you how to help a choking child or adult. Many free training classes are available. Check with your local hospital, city services, or Red Cross chapter.

4. **Clean out your medicine cabinet.**
   Make sure you have a complete, up-to-date first aid kit. Check the expiration dates on all your medications and throw away the ones that have expired. Some become more potent and others lose effectiveness, so don't take any chances. Make sure all your medications are stored where children can't reach them.

5. **Check your salad dressing.**
   According to the U.S. Department of Agriculture, the average American woman aged nineteen to fifty gets more fat from salad dressing than from any other food. Eating salad is a great way to get fiber and add veggies to your diet. Don't sabotage your efforts with a salad dressing high in fat or calories. Look for

some of the new salad "spritzer" dressings. They can add great flavor while keeping your calories as low as 10 calories per serving!

6. **Turn off your cell phone while driving.**
   You may be worried about the threat of cell phones and brain tumors (which has not been demonstrated by research), but the real threat from cell phones comes from using them while driving. One study showed that people who use cell phones while driving are four times as likely to have an accident that causes them injury. Using a hands-free phone doesn't decrease the risk and may even increase your chances of having an accident. So do yourself and others on the road a life-saving favor: when you get in the car—switch off your phone.

7. **Lower your blood pressure.**
   Try these five tips to lower your blood pressure: (1) Add thirty minutes of physical activity to your day. (2) Cut back on your alcohol. (3) Stop putting salt on your food. (4) Sit quietly and focus on your breathing for ten minutes each day. (5) Eat a banana (high in potassium) every day.

8. **Get a pneumonia vaccine.**
   This shot can protect you from the twenty-three strains of the pneumoccoccal bacteria that cause 88 percent of all cases of pneumonia in the United States. Getting the shot once gives you years of protection. People over sixty-five, who are most at risk of dying from pneumonia, and anyone who has a chronic condition or lower resistance to infection should talk with their doctor about getting vaccinated.

9. **Carry aspirin.**
   If you have a heart attack, quickly chewing an aspirin can save your life (chewing sends the aspirin into your bloodstream to inhibit clotting twice as quickly as swallowing it). Other painkillers such as Tylenol (acetaminophen), Motrin (ibuprofen), and others don't count—it must be *aspirin*. Buy some small travel packs and put one in your car, your purse, your gym bag, or your wallet—places you can get to quickly wherever you are.

10. **Step down your caffeine.**
    Too much caffeine can cause heart irregularities, anxiety, headaches, high blood pressure, insomnia, and more. But cutting back suddenly on caffeine can cause withdrawal effects such as headaches, fatigue, and irritability. Lower your caffeine gradually by cutting out half a cup of coffee every few days, mixing regular coffee with decaffeinated, and reducing other sources little by little.

11. **Practice safe sex no matter how old you are.**
    Practicing safe sex is essential to your health, even when the risk of pregnancy is no longer an issue. Sixty-one percent of older single adults say they're having unprotected sex. *Newsweek* reports that from 1990 to 2004, the number of AIDS cases in adults fifty and over grew sevenfold. Rates of gonorrhea and syphilis have increased by 55 percent as well. Older single adults are more sexually active than ever and should be equally responsible about protecting both themselves and their partners.

12. **Prevent colds.**
    During cold season, these four tips can keep you healthy: (1) Stay warm. Researchers now back up moms (finally) who have always known that getting a chill makes you more likely to get sick. (2) Wash your hands with soap and water. (3) Try not to touch your eyes, nose, and mouth (that's how the virus spreads). (4) Clean shared spaces like keyboards, phones, and office equipment.

13. **Drink tap water to prevent cavities.**
    In the 1960s, cities in the United States began to add fluoride to their water supplies to prevent cavities. And it worked—cavities became almost nonexistent. But in the last ten years, cavities have made a comeback, as we drink more bottled water, most of which don't have enough fluoride to prevent tooth decay. Get a reusable container and fill it from the tap rather than always resorting to bottled water, or buy bottled water that has added fluoride to protect those pearly whites.

14. **Learn to do breast (women) or testicular (men) exams.**
    A monthly self-exam is one of the ways to detect both breast

and testicular cancer in their earliest stages and can be done in the privacy of your home. Ask your doctor or visit www.tayloryourhealth.com/selfexams.html for instructions. Do the exam once a month. If you feel anything unusual, talk to your doctor right away—often it's nothing, but always get checked out.

15. **Know your kids' height and weight.**
Medication doses for kids (even over-the-counter) should be based on their weight rather than age, so make sure you weigh and measure your child at least every three months—more often for infants. Convert their weight to kilograms (see page 189) and write it down in their medical records so that you always have it handy in an emergency or when they're being given medication.

16. **Wear sunglasses.**
According to the American Optometric Association, the likelihood of developing eye diseases such as cataracts, light sensitivity, and nearsightedness significantly increases if you are in the sun for long hours without eye protection. Exposure to UV rays has also been linked to vision deterioration, growths on the surface of the eye, and cancer of the skin around the eyes and eyelids. And wearing sunglasses also has an effect on your appearance, reducing crow's feet and wrinkles around the eyes.

17. **Eat egg whites instead of whole eggs.**
At only 15 calories per egg, egg whites are almost like a free food! Compared to about 80 calories for a whole egg, egg whites are an easy way to save calories and help cut your cholesterol.

18. **Throw away your mercury thermometers.**
Many of us still have old-fashioned glass thermometers, which contain mercury. Surprisingly, these simple devices can be a threat to your family's health if they break. Mercury can cause tingling in the fingers and toes, numbness around the mouth, and tunnel vision. Long-term exposure can cause serious conditions. Buy an inexpensive mercury-free thermometer at any local drugstore and take your old mercury thermometers to a household hazardous waste-collection facility for disposal.

19. **Leave the elevator and walk up the stairs.**
    This trick can burn an extra hundred calories for every ten minutes of stair walking (up) you do. (Walking down the stairs burns less calories and can be harder on your knees and joints.)

20. **Add nutrition to your cooking.**
    Cooking with garlic, onions, basil, cumin, turmeric, black pepper, jalapeños (hot!), mustard, and cinnamon adds nutrients without extra calories.

21. **Fight chronic pain.**
    If you have chronic pain, talk with your doctor—don't just put up with it. These tips can also give you some relief: (1) Try to move as much as physically possible—muscle inactivity can worsen your pain (this does not apply to acute injuries). (2) Tune in to your body. Take five-minute breaks throughout your day to focus on breathing and relaxing. (3) Ask your doctor about doing nonimpact activities like swimming or bicycling, which can help circulation and help produce chemicals that aid in fighting pain.

22. **Count calories for one week.**
    Research shows that we underestimate how many calories we eat by as much as 75 percent! Write down everything you eat in a food log for one week. Count up your calories for each day. Take your target weight and multiply it by 15 to get a general estimate of your daily calorie allowance to maintain that weight. To lose weight, subtract 1,000 calories a day, writing down calories each day.

23. **Check your moles and skin.**
    Skin cancer is one of the most common forms of cancer and one of the most deadly, yet over half of all adults never check their skin. The good news is that it is also one of the easiest to detect and treat. Don't leave looking at your skin to the doc—you're a much better judge of changes and irritations (and the fact is, most doctors don't do it). Look for changes in color, size, or shape of moles and birthmarks or any sores that take more than a week or two to heal. For a detailed guide of what to check, visit www.tayloryourhealth.com/selfexams.html.

24. **Remove the drawstrings from kids' clothing.**
Children can get seriously injured and even suffocate if the drawstrings on necklines and hoods of their clothing get snagged on playground slides, school bus handrails, or doors. Cut waist and bottom drawstrings to three inches or less.

25. **Update your birth control.**
Several new forms of birth control are available, from contraceptive rings, patches, and injections to new forms of the Pill. Talk to your doctor about your reproductive needs and personal preferences to see if there's a new option you might prefer. Also, men, stay tuned: there's lots of research being done on a male contraceptive! Remember, most birth control methods don't protect against disease, so talk to your doctor about what works best.

26. **Take a fish oil capsule every day.**
Fish oil contains powerful omega-3 fatty acids that help lower bad cholesterol. The American Heart Association recommends a daily fish oil capsule, especially if you tend to have high levels of triglycerides, which can put you at risk for having a sudden heart attack.

27. **Go over your medications with your doctor.**
Make a list of all the medications you take, including prescription, over-the-counter, supplements, and even vitamins. Review it with your doctor at your next visit (keep the list handy for emergencies, too). He can check for any possible interactions and evaluate how well the medications are working. Doctors will sometimes eliminate one or two drugs that you no longer need.

28. **Update your tetanus booster.**
Tetanus, commonly called lockjaw, is a completely preventable but potentially fatal disease. Tetanus bacteria are commonly found in dirt, soil, and manure—one-third of tetanus infections occur during gardening. You might think that shots are just for kids, but tetanus protection lasts only about ten years and 53 percent of Americans over twenty aren't protected. Check when you had your last vaccine and get a booster if it's been more than ten years.

29. **Protect the privacy of your medical records.**
You expect privacy when it comes to your health information, but that's not always the case. Today any number of organizations have access to your most private information, which can be used inappropriately. Take these steps to protect your health information: (1) Don't put personal health information online. (2) Ask your doctor whom he releases your information to and for what purposes. (3) Don't sign blanket disclosure forms agreeing to the release of your medical records.

30. **Beware of iguanas.**
Ownership of reptile pets has increased more than twenty-eight-fold since 1986 in the United States, with the majority being iguanas. While fun to watch, these creatures cause thousands of cases of salmonella poisoning each year and sometimes even death. Make sure you and any children who come into contact with iguanas, snakes, and other reptiles wash your hands thoroughly with soap and water. Experts recommend not keeping these pets if you have small children in your household.

31. **Plant your family tree.**
Make a family health tree listing relatives on both sides, including your mother, father, sisters, brothers, aunts, uncles, and grandparents. List any health conditions you're aware of and the cause of death for relatives who are no longer living. Pay particular attention to relatives who passed away at a young age. Review the list with your doctor at your next visit to help her figure out what tests or preventive measures you should have.

32. **Last call for alcohol.**
Cutting back on the amount of alcohol you drink can have lots of benefits: improving your heart health, lowering your blood pressure, eliminating impotence (men), reducing your cancer risk, and reducing the risk of stroke, not to mention just generally making you feel better. A couple of drinks a day doesn't seem to have a bad effect on your health (and may even be beneficial in some ways), but moderation is the key. And be sure to always ask yourself, Am I drinking because I want to or because I need to?

33. **Clean out your car.**
Loose objects can become dangerous projectiles in your car if you stop suddenly or have an accident. Something as seemingly harmless as a cell phone can cause a skull fracture or other life-threatening injury. If you have a cargo area, use a cargo net or tie down any items, and be sure everyone is belted in.

34. **Get a diabetes test.**
Millions of Americans have type 2 diabetes and don't know it. Millions more have prediabetes—blood sugar levels above normal, but not in the diabetes range. The good news is that if you have type 2 diabetes and are diagnosed early enough, you can probably control your condition just with diet and exercise. If you are in the prediabetes range, now is the time to improve your habits to get your blood sugar levels down to normal.

35. **Save money on prescription drugs.**
The cost for drugs keeps taking a bigger bite out of your health care budget. These tips can save you money on prescription drugs: (1) Ask your doctor for free samples. (2) Shop around for the lowest price. Check different pharmacies, mail order, and online. (3) Look for patient-assistance programs offered by drug manufacturers. Check the Partnership for Prescription Assistance Web site www.pparx.org or call 888-477-2669 for help.

36. **Go to the dentist.**
It's best to visit your dentist every six months, but don't go longer than a year without a checkup. It's not just a beautiful smile—dental infections and gum disease can affect your health, even leading to heart disease. If you avoid the dentist, try these tactics to make you more comfortable: (1) Look for a dentist who practices "pain-free" dentistry. (2) Take an aspirin an hour before your visit to combat any discomfort. (3) Talk with your dentist before any procedure about the pain management techniques she will use. (4) Agree on a hand signal with the dentist or assistants that will let them know you are in pain and want the procedure to stop.

37. **Drink more water.**
Don't just think about it, do it. Water is the best substance you

can put into your body. Make a list of the eight times during the day you will drink a glass of water and check them off each day. (Sodas, coffee, and other drinks don't count.)

38. **Give your home a safety checkup.**
A third of all injuries happen in the home. Give your home a safety checkup at least once a year. Some items to check: cords (tripping hazard), medication storage (away from children), rugs (for slipping and tripping), working smoke detectors, outlets (for electrical fire hazards), and space heaters (for fire hazard). Be sure that everyone knows how to get out of the house in case of a fire or emergency. To create a personalized home safety checklist, visit www.homesafetycouncil.org.

39. **Eat peanut butter.**
High in vitamin E and antioxidants, peanut butter appears to protect against heart disease and helps to control weight. It offers a lot of nutrition for the calories, without containing a high level of saturated fats (the bad kind). The government requires all peanut butter to be made from 90 percent peanuts, so you don't have to worry about additives or a lot of other ingredients. Always check for peanut allergies before eating or serving it.

40. **Eat one new fruit or vegetable a day for a week.**
There's lots of fruits or vegetables out there that you probably haven't tried. To spice up your diet, try a different one every day for a week. Add those you like to your diet on a permanent basis. You know you can't go wrong adding more fruits and veggies to your daily diet.

41. **Wear sunscreen on your lips.**
Lip cancer is the most common form of oral cancer and is caused most often by unprotected sun exposure. So don't forget those luscious lips when applying sunscreen. Check your lip balm to make sure it has SPF protection—use zinc oxide if you're going to be in direct sunlight for a long time.

42. **Count your steps.**
Buy an inexpensive pedometer and wear it for a week to count your steps. Try to work up to 10,000 steps, about five miles, a day. Unless you have a walking-intensive job like a nurse or mail

carrier, you'll probably have to add a thirty-minute walk to your day to get up to that number.

43. **Learn how to give yourself the Heimlich maneuver.**
    If you are alone and begin to choke, knowing how to give yourself the Heimlich maneuver can save your life. Press your upper abdomen (just below the ribs) forcefully against the back of a chair, a table, a sink, or a railing. Repeat until air is forced through your airway and the food you are choking on is expelled.

44. **Make a travel health kit.**
    One in four travelers experiences an illness or injury, so be prepared. Your kit should include: (1) a portable version of your critical health information (visit www.tayloryourhealth.com for info on Pocket Health Organizers), (2) enough medications to cover your trip, plus an extra week's supply, (3) a list of doctors and hospitals in the areas you're traveling through and to (especially important if you manage a chronic health condition), and (4) a mini first-aid kit containing pain relievers, antidiarrheal tablets, motion sickness pills, antibacterial cream, antiseptic, bandages, and other emergency supplies.

45. **Keep your mind sharp.**
    When it comes to your brain, you truly use it or lose it. Try these tips to keep you on top of your game: (1) Eat brain foods, including fish, green veggies, grape juice, and beans. (2) Listen to music to stimulate various parts of your brain. (3) Be physically active. This will keep oxygen flowing to your brain. (4) Socialize. Meeting new people stimulates your memory and keeps you engaged. (5) Fall in love—with a person, a pet, a child, or a new hobby. Feelings of happiness and love release chemicals that stimulate the brain, so find yourself someone to love.

46. **Drink tea, wonderful tea.**
    Tea is being touted as a wonder drink, and it's no wonder. Some doctors say it is the single best thing you can add to your diet to keep illness at bay, including preventing cancer and heart disease. In just one study (and there are lots), women age fifty-five or older who drank one cup of black tea a day were 54 percent

less likely to have severely clogged arteries, which can lead to heart attack and stroke. The more tea they drank, the more their risk went down. And since tea has very few calories, you're getting all the benefits while watching your weight.

47. **Get your eyes checked.**
    Children and everyone over forty should have their eyes checked every two years—every year if you're over sixty-five. Eye problems can develop slowly, but if you wait until your vision is affected, it may be too late to get the best treatment. Get your eyes checked more frequently if you start having vision problems or experience headaches when reading or watching TV.

48. **Round out your physical activity.**
    Make sure your activity plan includes the big three: aerobics (exercising your heart), strength (for muscles), and stretching (to keep you flexible). Find a variety of activities that fit into your everyday life that help you hit all the categories.

49. **Learn the warning signs of a heart attack.**
    Thousands of people die each year because they did not get fast enough treatment for a heart attack. Learn to recognize the symptoms and *get immediate treatment*. Some of the signs can include chest pains or tightness and pain radiating down the arms (especially left), dizziness, nausea, trouble breathing, and sudden sweating. If you have had a heart attack before, it's likely you will not have chest pain. If you have dizziness or difficulty catching your breath, call 9-1-1 or go to the closest ER.

50. **Get the most from your insurance plan.**
    You're paying for coverage, so make sure you understand your plan and what you're eligible for. Understand your copayments, what your yearly deductible is (the amount you have to pay before benefits kick in), and what preventive health care the plan covers at a low cost or for free. Take advantage of these services to keep yourself healthy and your health care costs down.

51. **See your doctor quarterly.**
    With the average doctor's visit clocking in at eleven minutes, it's nearly impossible for you and your doctor to cover all your health issues and questions, let alone develop a prevention plan,

at a once-yearly visit. You could even schedule quarterly check-ups to discuss different issues. For example, spring (heart health), summer (skin check), fall (cancer review), winter (diet and exercise). Your doctor will get to know you better, and you'll stop feeling rushed at each visit.

52. **Give yourself a break.**
Take a break from your health. There may be habits that stuck and habits that stunk, but give yourself a pat on the back for all you've accomplished in the last fifty-two weeks and *celebrate*! Remember, the important thing is to make changes where you can. Your health is twenty-four hours a day, 365 days a year. You won't always make healthy choices, but even a few changes will help you see a big difference. The best health tip I can give you is . . .

Live, Laugh, Love.
Fifty-two weeks a year.

Appendix
Health Care Glossary

Below are definitions to help you understand what your doctors are saying, choose people and facilities that are right for you, and find the health care resources you need.

Medical Specialties

Allergist Allergies and asthma

Anesthesiology Administration of anesthesia for surgery

Cardiology Heart

Cardiothoracic surgery Heart and chest surgery

Dermatology Skin

Emergency medicine Emergency room care

Endocrinology Endocrine glands such as diabetes or thyroid disorders

Family practice General medicine, pediatrics, mental health, and OB/GYN

Gastroenterology Digestive system (stomach and intestines)

General practice General patient care and coordinates care

Genetics Hereditary diseases

Geriatrics Senior health

Hematology Blood disease and disorders

Immunology Immune system

Infectious diseases Diseases spread through viruses or bacteria

Internal medicine Nonsurgical treatment of adults

Nephrology Kidneys

Neurology Nervous system (the brain and spinal cord)

Neurosurgery Brain and spinal cord surgery

Obstetrics Pregnancy and birth

Oncology Cancer

Ophthalmology Eyes

Orthopedics Bones and ligaments

Otorhinolaryngology Ear, nose, and throat (ENT)

Pathology Laboratory study of tissues

Pediatrics Babies, children, and adolescents

Pharmacology Drugs and medication

Podiatry Feet

Psychiatry Mental and emotional disorders

Pulmonology Lungs

Radiology Use of X-rays to diagnose and treat diseases

Rheumatology Joints, muscles, and bones

Toxicology Poisonous substances and their antidotes

Urology Urinary system and male reproductive system

Health Care Professionals

Audiologist Works in the detection and treatment of hearing problems.

Chiropractor Realigns the spine through physical manipulation.

Dietitian Develops diets to meet patients' specific requirements, including weight loss, diabetes, and other conditions.

Emergency Medical Technician (EMT) Trained in emergency life support and the care and transport of the ill and injured to hospitals. Also called paramedic.

Home health aide Provides health care in the home for those unable to fully care for themselves, including dressing, bathing, eating, and simple nursing tasks such as changing bandages and medication assistance.

Laboratory technician Performs tests on blood, urine, and other substances to help in the diagnosis and treatment of illness and injury.

Midwife Assists in the delivery of babies, helps women in labor, and provides prenatal care.

Nurse practitioner Provides high-level nursing services under the guidance of a physician, including diagnosing conditions, prescribing medications (only in some states), taking health histories, and coordinating patients' overall care.

Nurse's aide Provides simple nursing tasks in hospitals, including feeding, bathing, and moving patients. Because of the current shortage of nurses, in some hospitals, aides may perform tasks normally performed by nurses, including giving injections, drawing blood, and reading monitoring devices.

Occupational therapist Helps those who are injured or disabled regain their ability to function and carry out everyday tasks.

Optician Grinds and fits eyeglasses and contact lenses.

Optometrist Performs vision tests and writes prescriptions for eyeglasses and contact lenses.

Physical therapist Uses techniques such as exercise and massage to help patients regain lost physical functions due to illness or injury.

Physician's assistant Works under a physician's supervision to examine patients and provide basic health services and diagnoses.

Psychologist Uses counseling and therapy to treat mental health issues.

Radiology technician Takes and develops X-rays, CT scans, and other tests using radiation.

Respiration therapist Improves breathing ability and capacity using respirators and other devices.

Speech therapist Treats disorders and injuries that affect speech.

Types of Hospitals

When scheduling a surgery or choosing a surgeon, you should consider what type of hospital would be the best place to have your surgery. It's important to select a hospital that is accredited and also has the right equipment, staff, and experience for your specific surgical procedure.

Community hospitals Smaller hospitals that serve the medical needs of local communities, focusing on patient care. This can be a good choice for minor surgeries when you want personalized, comfortable care at a convenient location. They can also be a great resource for community health services such as diabetes management instruction, prenatal classes, CPR training, and other health support services.

Major academic medical centers These facilities provide the majority of care for people with complex medical conditions. Typically affiliated with a medical school, these hospitals also train doctors and other health care professionals and conduct medical research. This is where you want to go if your condition would benefit from the latest medical technologies and cutting-edge therapies. You can also look here for clinical trials that may give you access to research treatments not yet available to the general population. You should be aware that interns, residents, and other staff-in-training will be a large part of your medical care.

Public hospitals Public hospitals are owned by the government and thus usually provide care regardless of a patient's ability to pay. This doesn't mean they provide substandard care. On the contrary, they are often affiliated with medical schools and serve as teaching and research hospitals. Again, it's important to check the accreditation, rating, and local reputation of any hospital before you go there for care.

Rehabilitation centers If your surgery requires a long recuperation period, typically you will be transferred to one of these facilities once your condition has stabilized. These facilities concentrate on helping patients adjust to and compensate for physical changes and regain independence. The rehabilitation staff may include psychiatrists, physicians, occupational therapists, nurses, social workers, and others who can help you, depending on your individual needs. Look for a well-equipped facility with experienced staff and up-to-date equipment.

Specialty centers Hospitals that are focused on treating a specific type of condition (such as cancer, vision, spine) or group of people (women, children) are good to use once you have a firm diagnosis. They can also have higher-end, specialized equipment and doctors geared directly toward your specific condition. Make sure they are accredited, have a good reputation in the medical community, and have the staff and facilities to treat your condition. They are also usually not the best resource for general overall care, since they focus on one or more specialties.

Mental Health Professionals

Certified alcohol and drug abuse counselor Trained in alcohol and drug abuse. Trained to diagnose abuse issues and offer counseling in both an individual and a group setting. Qualifications: state license.

Certified Mental Health Counselor (CMHC) Master's degree and several years of supervised clinical work experience. Qualifications: certification by the National Academy of Certified Clinical Mental Health Counselors.

Child psychiatrist Medical doctor with training in the diagnosis and treatment of emotional and behavioral issues in children. Child psychiatrists are authorized to prescribe medications. Qualifications: state medical license and certification by the American Board of Psychiatry and Neurology.

Licensed Clinical Social Worker (LCSW) Master's degree in social work. Often employed by government agencies or hospitals to offer assistance with child abuse, family, and health issues. Qualifications: state license; possibly member of Academy of Certified Social Workers.

Licensed Professional Counselor (LPC) Master's degree in psychology, counseling, or related field. Provides individual or group counseling. Qualifications: state license.

Marriage, Family, and Child Counselor (MFCC) Usually have a master's degree (but some states require only a bachelor's degree) and hundreds to thousands of hours of counseling experience. Qualifications: state license.

Pastoral counselor Clergy with training in clinical pastoral education. Qualifications: certification from American Association of Pastoral Counselors.

Psychiatric nurse Registered nurse (RN) with a master's degree, trained to assess mental and physical illness. May provide counseling. In some states, it is legal for a psychiatric nurse to prescribe medicine. Qualifications: certification, state license.

Psychiatrist Medical doctor trained in the diagnosis and treatment of mental and emotional conditions. Authorized to prescribe medications. Most focus on medication therapy, although a few do psychotherapy as well. Qualifications: state medical license and certification by the American Board of Psychiatry and Neurology.

Psychologist Doctorate from an accredited graduate program in psychology and two or more years of supervised work experience, usually focused on psychotherapy. Often uses tests such as IQ tests, personality tests, and career tests. Cannot prescribe medicines in most states. Qualifications: state license.

Psychotherapist General term used to refer to those who provide mental health counseling. May refer to someone with or without specialized training or a degree.

School psychologist Most school psychologists have a doctorate degree. Trained to help students with school and personal issues such as learning disabilities, behavior issues, and family issues. Provide therapy only as it relates to helping students. Qualifications: state license.

Mental Health Therapies

There are many different types of mental health therapies. Mental health professionals may utilize different types of therapies depending on their experience, personal preference, and patient needs. It's important to ask what type of therapies they use and understand them so that you know you will be comfortable and the therapy can be effective. If you don't like the therapy, tell your counselor or doctor or find someone else who uses a method that you prefer. A few of the main types are listed here.

Behavioral therapy Structured and goal-oriented therapy that focuses on what you are doing now and how you can change your behavior. May use biofeedback, aversion, role-playing, and self-monitoring.

Cognitive behavioral therapy Short-term therapy (usually around sixteen sessions) that helps you identify and correct unhelpful or destructive thinking patterns, replacing these with more realistic and helpful ones. Homework helps you focus on how you behave now and develop strategies for positive thinking.

Family or couples therapy Therapy provided to both members of a couple or members of a family together to help them improve their relationship and function better together. Works on communication, positive behaviors, and mutual support. May include role-playing and individual counseling, as well.

Group therapy A small number of people meet regularly with a therapist. Some groups are general and others are focused on a specific issue like anger management. Groups may be short-term or ongoing. Boundaries are set by the therapist, but members provide one another with insight and feedback.

Medication therapy The use of prescription medicines to treat mental conditions and improve your mental well-being. There are many types of psychiatric medications, so your doctor must first identify your condition in order to prescribe the proper medication. Often combined with talk therapy to most effectively help address your emotional needs.

Movement/Art/Music therapy Therapies include the use of dance, art, or music to express emotions. Can be especially effective for children or others who may have difficulty expressing emotions in traditional therapy methods.

Pastoral therapy Some people prefer to seek therapy from their pastor, rabbi, or other faith-based counselors. Typically incorporates aspects of psychotherapy with prayer and spirituality to address mental and emotional issues.

Play therapy Allows children to act out their problems with toys and games. Play therapists can help a child feel more confident and less fearful.

Psychoanalysis Developed by Freud, this therapy helps you uncover things from your past that may be affecting your thoughts, moods, emotions, and behaviors. It often takes years to discover and address issues.

Talk therapy Used to describe therapy methods where the emphasis is on the patient talking to the therapist to express and resolve issues.

Tests and Screenings

Angiography Dye is injected into arteries to identify blockages.

Arthroscopy A tube is inserted into a joint to view or biopsy.

Barium enema Fluid containing barium dye is introduced into your colon to check for tumors, polyps, or gastrointestinal problems.

Biopsy Small sample of tissue or fluid is removed, either surgically or with a needle, for further testing.

Blood glucose Blood test that determines the amount of sugar (glucose) in your blood to indicate whether you may have diabetes.

Bone density Measures the density of bones using X-rays.

Bone marrow aspiration and biopsy A needle is used to obtain a sample of bone marrow—the soft tissue inside your bones—to diagnose blood disorders, severe anemia, cancers, and other diseases.

Bronchoscopy A thin, flexible tube passed through the nose to allow a physician to check for tumors, bleeding, blockages, and other lung or throat abnormalities.

Colonoscopy A thin, flexible tube passed through the anus, rectum, and intestine to allow a physician to check for signs of disease, obtain tissue samples, or remove polyps.

Colposcopy A thin, flexible tube inserted into the vagina to allow a physician to inspect the cervix and vagina for tumors or other abnormalities.

CT scan (Computerizd tomography) Often called a CAT scan. Imaging test that uses multiple X-ray images to construct two-dimensional images of organs or regions of the body.

Cystoscopy A tube inserted into the bladder to allow a physician to inspect the bladder for abnormalities or blockages.

Digital rectal exam A physician inserts a gloved finger into the rectum to check for enlargements, bumps, and other abnormalities, typically to aid in detection of prostate cancer in men.

EKG (Electrocardiography) The electrical activity of the heart is monitored through small metal sensors placed on your chest. Used to detect heart attacks, coronary artery blockages, and other heart abnormalities.

ERCP (Endoscopic retrograde cholangiopancreatography) A thin, flexible, lighted tube is inserted through your mouth into your digestive tract, where dye is used to detect pancreatic cancer, bile duct obstructions, and other abnormalities of the pancreas.

Fecal blood occult Stool samples are analyzed for small amounts of blood that might indicate internal bleeding, cancer, or other conditions.

Glaucoma screening (Tonometry) Measures the fluid pressure within the eye by applying gentle pressure on the cornea.

IVP (Intravenous pyelography) Dye is injected into a vein in your arm while X-rays are taken as the dye flows through the kidneys, ureters, and bladder to locate kidney stones, tumors, infections, or other urinary conditions.

Laryngoscopy A thin, flexible viewing tube is passed through the nose to allow a physician to inspect the throat, nose, and larynx for lesions or signs of cancer or to obtain tissue samples.

Mammogram X-rays are passed through the breast to detect tumors, cysts, and other abnormalities.

MRI (Magnetic resonance imaging) Imaging test that uses radio wave signals to compose detailed, cross-section views of organs and regions of your body.

Myelography Dye is injected into the space around your spinal cord and brain and X-rays are used to detect tumors, herniated disks, nerve injuries, and other conditions and abnormalities.

Pap smear For women, a sample of cells scraped from your cervix is tested to reveal precancerous and cancerous conditions.

Pelvic exam For women, a physician inspects your reproductive organs to detect any abnormalities or conditions.

Prostate exam See **digital rectal exam**.

PSA blood test Used to detect elevated levels of PSA (prostate-specific antigen) as a possible sign of prostate cancer or other prostate infections.

Sigmoidoscopy A flexible, lighted viewing tube is passed through the anus, rectum, and colon to allow a physician to check for tumors or signs of colorectal cancer and other conditions.

Snellen test Commonly used eye test that has you look at a chart with various-size letters to determine how well you see objects and assigns a number rating to each eye (20/20 vision, for example).

Spinal tap (Lumbar puncture) A thin needle is inserted into your spinal column to measure pressure and obtain a fluid sample.

Tuberculosis skin test A tuberculin antigen is injected into the skin of your forearm. If you have been exposed to tuberculosis, there will be a reaction at the injection site.

Ultrasound Sound waves are used to compose a two-dimensional picture of a fetus, organ, or region of the body. Most commonly used on pregnant women to view the fetus, but also used quite often to look at other organs for abnormalities.

Upper GI (Upper gastrointestinal) After drinking a liquid dye, X-rays are taken of your esophagus, stomach, and upper intestine to detect abnormalities.

Urinalysis Various tests performed on a urine sample to detect kidney disorders, urinary tract infections, and other conditions.

Index